Drinking in Victorian and Edwardian Britain

Thora Hands

Drinking in Victorian and Edwardian Britain

Beyond the Spectre of the Drunkard

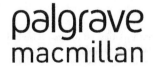

Thora Hands
Social Sciences
City of Glasgow College
Glasgow, UK

ISBN 978-3-319-92963-7   ISBN 978-3-319-92964-4   (eBook)
https://doi.org/10.1007/978-3-319-92964-4

Library of Congress Control Number: 2018943635

Cover image: © Thora Hands

Printed on acid-free paper

This Palgrave Macmillan imprint is published by the registered company Springer
International Publishing AG part of Springer Nature
The registered company address is: Gewerbestrasse 11, 6330 Cham, Switzerland

For Corky

PREFACE

> It is not a dark secret, nor is it difficult to perceive, that the established
> intellectual research disciplines ... when they turned their attention to
> alcohol, man and society focused upon the painful aspects. They studied
> 'drinks' not drinkers; intoxication rather than drinking; the awful sequels
> of alcohol ingestion, not the usual. Studies of the causes of alcoholism for
> example, are legion, but studies of the causes of drinking are rare'[1]

My background is in social sciences and next to history, sociology is my
second great interest. So before embarking on historical research for
my thesis, my Ph.D. supervisor Jim Mills drew my attention to a collection of sociological and anthropological studies on alcohol and drinking
behaviour. The quote above is from Selden Bacon, an American sociologist writing in the 1970s on the limitations of the problem framework
within alcohol studies. Bacon and other sociologists, such as Harry
Levine, were critical of scientific approaches that focused primarily on
the issue of pathology because they felt that these studies simply miss
the point of alcohol consumption.[2] Put simply, most people who drink
alcohol are not alcoholics and therefore it seems illogical to focus almost
exclusively on that aspect of drinking behaviour.

Levine links the emergence of the pathological framework to a 'temperance culture' in which alcohol is viewed as a problem or social evil. In
countries like Britain, this sort of attitude has prevailed for a long time—
right back to the nineteenth century in fact.[3] More recently, the idea
of a temperance culture has a particular resonance because my country,

Scotland, passed a law that will introduce minimum unit pricing on alcoholic drinks. This is a population-wide measure to tackle the health and social problems associated with alcohol consumption. Whether it will make any kind of decisive impact on drinking behaviour is yet to be seen, but it is a measure that affects all alcohol consumers in Scotland and it is based upon the premise that alcohol is a social problem.

The sociologist in me questions the limitations of the problem framework because it fails to account for human agency or for the complexities of alcohol production and consumption. This not only limits our understanding of drinking behaviour but it also impacts upon the majority of alcohol consumers. I'm not only talking about present-day drinkers in Scotland but also those in the past for whom alcohol was not a problem but a substance that held pleasure and meaning. As Bacon said, the ordinary aspects of alcohol have never really grabbed the limelight and that also applies to the historical record. The Victorian period was the original temperance culture, where alcohol and drunkenness were constructed as social and moral problems and that is why it offered the perfect place to start digging around for a different side to the story.

Thora Hands

NOTES

1. Bacon S. 1979. 'Alcohol Research Policy: The Need for an Independent Phenomenologically Oriented Field of Studies': *Journal of Studies of Alcohol*: Volume 8:2: p. 26
2. Levine H. 1991. 'The Promise and Problems of Alcohol Sociology', in (ed.) Roman P. M. *Alcohol: The Development of Sociological Perspectives on Use and Abuse*: New Jersey: Rutgers Centre of Alcohol Studies.
3. Ibid.: p. 106.

ACKNOWLEDGEMENTS

This book marks a journey that began ten years ago when I frantically scribbled a one-page essay to gain entry to a social sciences college course and ended when I received my doctorate in history. I hope that the journey is not yet over but for that stage at least, I have to thank the many people who helped me along the way.

In my new role as a college lecturer, I now know just how committed and inspiring my own lecturers were and without the help and support of Lynn Dickie, Iain MacPherson and Jennifer Gemmell of the former Langside College, I would not have made it on to the degree programme at Glasgow Caledonian University. The jump from degree to Masters involved a mix of good luck in finding the Girgenti records at the Mitchell library (so thank you drunken Edwardian women!) and further good fortune in having a wonderful supervisor, Dr. Janet Greenlees, who showed no end of patience and encouragement in guiding me on to the Ph.D. This book is based on my doctoral thesis and for that, I have to thank my Ph.D. supervisors Professor Jim Mills and Professor Matt Smith of Strathclyde University for their help and support. I would also like to thank the Faculty of Education and Society at City of Glasgow College for supporting the publication of this book.

I owe a great debt of gratitude to The Wellcome Trust for funding my Doctoral research project titled 'Reframing Drink and the Victorians: The Consumption of Alcohol in Britain 1869–1914' (reference no. 099357/Z/12/Z). This allowed me to visit wonderful archives that contained fascinating material. I was awed by the sheer volume and diversity of the Diageo archive near Stirling and I have to thank the generosity and patience of the archivists there. I also owe many thanks to the archivists at The Athenaeum and The Reform Clubs in London for showing such interest in my research and allowing me to sift through their club records to uncover a wealth of material. I spent many happy days in the National Brewing Archive in Burton-upon-Trent and thank the archivists for their knowledge and guidance.

Some of the best moments of my Ph.D. were at the conferences hosted by The Alcohol and Drug History Society. I have rarely spent time with a bunch of academics who are as supportive and generous with their time and knowledge and are generally just good fun to be around. I owe particular thanks to Dr. Iain Smith for being such a good travelling companion; to David Fahey for sharing his mighty knowledge of British alcohol history and to Dan Malleck for being an all-round good guy.

My biggest thanks go to my mum Kathy and to my partner Andy for their support and most importantly, for pouring wine or mixing margaritas as and when necessary. My kids—Dan, Lewi, Peter and Beth have been with me throughout this journey. They have grown up with a mum often chained to a desk piled high with books, or packing a case to go off on research and they just rolled with it, as kids do, but they should know that I appreciate the time they gave me and that they have my love, always.

CONTENTS

LIST OF FIGURES

CHAPTER 1

Introduction: Reframing Drink and the Victorians

The Victorians liked to drink and they lived in a society geared towards alcohol consumption. In the great industrial cities of Britain, there was almost no escaping the beer houses; gin palaces; refreshment rooms; restaurants; theatres; music halls; vaults; dram shops; oyster bars; private clubs and public houses that served a dizzying array of alcoholic drinks to suit people from all walks of life. Drinking went on from dawn till dusk and on into the wee small hours so we know that many people liked to drink. Yet we know very little about their reasons for doing so because the issue of drunkenness has cast a long shadow over the majority of alcohol consumers. In reframing drink and the Victorians, this book looks deeper than the problems of alcohol, to investigate the reasons why people drank it in the first place. It picks up where Brian Harrison's study of the Victorian temperance movement ended and surveys the period from 1869, when the state began to take more control of alcohol regulation and licensing, up until 1914 when wartime regulations were imposed on alcohol sale and consumption.[1] Harrison's study ended just at the point when the expansion and consolidation of the alcohol industry gave consumers more choice than ever in the types of alcoholic drinks they consumed and in the types of drinking places they frequented. Alcohol became a mass-produced commodity available to an expanding consumer market and this led to heightened political, moral and medical concerns about the problems associated with drinking and drunkenness across towns and cities in Britain.

© The Author(s) 2018
T. Hands, *Drinking in Victorian and Edwardian Britain*,
https://doi.org/10.1007/978-3-319-92964-4_1

1

Many questions about drink and the Victorians remain unanswered but the most pressing relate to how and why the majority of people carried on drinking through a period when it was increasingly difficult to do so in a socially acceptable way. The clues to answering this question lie partly in the substance itself. Alcohol is and was a legal intoxicant that derives its usage and meaning from the social and cultural context in which it is consumed. People share a complex relationship with alcohol that spans time and place but importantly, it is a relationship that involves the agency of consumers. This is why the story of drink in late Victorian and Edwardian Britain resonates today. We live in the consumer society that emerged from late nineteenth century industrial capitalism. The technological advances, production and advertising techniques developed during this time not only turned alcohol into a mass-produced commodity but also gave life to the idea of the consumer. People's drinking behaviour may have been shaped and constrained within a political, medical and moral framework but legislation and public health initiatives only went so far to control drinking behaviour within a political and economic system geared up for mass production and consumption. This is our current dilemma with alcohol and it stems from the late Victorian period. History has shown that it does not matter how often or to what extent alcohol consumption has been problematised or prohibited—people still continue to drink. Therefore, the key to understanding drinking behaviour is to try and understand why people drink. In this regard, the late Victorian period offers the perfect place to start.

Ronald Weir argues that the biggest demon facing the government and the drink trade in Victorian Britain was the 'spectre of the drunkard' which drove the political campaigns of the Temperance movement, shaped legislation and pushed the drink trade into a defensive position.[2] Early in the century, medical interest in the issue of drunkenness led to the development of the disease concept of inebriety which gained popularity in the 1870s as a means of diagnosing and medically treating heavy drinking and drug use. The British Society for the Study of Inebriety was formed in 1884 by a group of doctors and politicians who campaigned for legislation to legally detain and medically treat inebriates. This resulted in the passing of The Inebriates Act in 1898.[3]

Moral and medical concerns about drunkenness drove political campaigns to reform the licensing system in Britain and in the 1860s the 'drink question' topped party political agendas as a means to win over the electorate. The Liberal Party was broadly aligned with the pro-temperance campaigns that sought radical reforms of the licensing system. While in contrast, the Conservative Party sided more with the drink trade in aiming to maintain the status quo and protect the rights of alcohol producers, retailers and consumers.[4] In response to the tighter alcohol regulations imposed by the 1869 and 1872 Licensing Acts, the drink trade consolidated its efforts to mount political opposition that would challenge legislation and defend the right to buy and consume alcoholic drinks.[5] At the turn of the century, the stakes were high in the political 'battle' between the state and the drink trade, with the trade facing the prospect of a slow demise and the government facing the wrath of the drinking, pub-going electorate. The main source of debate was over the extent to which the state could legitimately interfere in a private enterprise. The trade was incensed by proposals to directly limit the numbers of pubs; grant more powers to local authorities to limit pub licenses within their districts and remove the profit from selling alcohol by establishing state and local authority run pubs. The 1904 Licensing Act passed by the Conservative government allowed for a reduction in licenses and compensation for the trade. However, as James Nicholls notes, the perceived weakness of this act fundamentally shifted the debate to one of direct state control over the drink trade which seemed unlikely until the outbreak of war in 1914 when the government was forced to take more direct action.[6]

Despite the problems of alcohol, it remained a legal intoxicant and in a recent study, Virginia Berridge considered the reasons why alcohol, unlike other narcotic substances remained legal in Britain. She argues that during the nineteenth century, temperance ideology and the economics of alcohol production were crucial in altering social, cultural and political attitudes towards alcohol.[7] The consolidation and expansion of the drink trade not only meant that alcohol became a standardised commodity produced for a mass market but it also increased the political influence of the drink trade. In short, the revenue generated from alcohol sales held its own political value.[8] Therein lies the issue with alcohol: moral and medical concerns about drinking fit uneasily within a capitalist system geared up to cater to an expanding consumer market. Attitudes towards alcohol may have changed but its commodity value remained solid.

Yet this commodity value was largely dependent upon the ability of the drink trade to generate and expand the market for alcohol. This was achieved through the invention of new technology that revolutionised the practices of brewers and distillers and allowed for the mass production of beers and spirits. Mid-century improvements in shipping and the expansion of the railways meant that alcohol producers could build the domestic and foreign markets for their products. British imperialism also provided a back-bone for trade by creating military and colonial outlets for alcoholic products. The retail trade expanded after the passing of The 1860 Wine and Refreshment Houses Act which was intended to promote the more 'civilised' habit of wine drinking by allowing the sale of wine and spirits within a wider range of premises. This stimulated the retail trade and led to the growth of refreshment rooms and licensed grocers. It also led to the success of businesses such as The Victoria Wine Company, a retail chain that catered to the more affluent urban middle classes.[9] This all added up to more choice in what people could drink and where they could drink. Most importantly, Victorians continued to step through the pub door even when the moral, political and medical tide began to turn against alcohol. We know that there was widespread concern about public drunkenness and that efforts were made to tackle this problem. We also know that drunkenness was constructed in religious, political and medical discourse as a moral failing; a medical problem; a source of social and financial ruin; the root of crime and deviance. Yet people still drank alcohol and we really know very little about their reasons for doing so.

BEYOND THE SPECTRE OF THE DRUNKARD

One of the ways of looking deeper than the problems of drink is to consider the agency of alcohol consumers. This type of analysis has been used in a number of social and cultural histories of alcohol and other intoxicants.[10] In a study of Mexican drinking culture, Tim Mitchell views drinkers as rational actors and not 'mere pawns somehow incapable of noticing alcohol's dark side'. He believes that the clues to uncovering people's motivations and drinking behaviour lie at the deeper cultural level.[11] In a study of cigarette smoking in America, Richard Klein claims that the 'dark, dangerous and sublime' qualities of cigarettes have been erased in a climate of demonization. He argues that cigarettes and smoking have a rich and diverse cultural history that can be explored and understood through a variety of cultural texts without reference to health risks, harm or addiction.[12] This is a useful methodology for looking at evidence of drinking behaviour because it negates the constant need to moralise drinking in the past. For the majority of alcohol consumers, drinking and getting drunk were choices—wilful acts involving the consumption of an intoxicant that held pleasure and meaning. This cannot be ignored or sidestepped by a moralising analysis. To do so would be to deny agency to consumers and disregard the social and cultural significance of a popular legal intoxicant.[13]

Looking beyond the problem framework also requires an understanding of the motives of alcohol producers and consumers. Sociological theories of consumption provide insights into how certain social groups cultivated tastes for particular drinks and how and why needs and desires for specific drinks were generated. Thorstein Veblen's ideas about conspicuous consumption prove useful in considering the drinking behaviour of the middle and upper classes. Veblen argues that the overt display of wealth was one way that the Victorian upper classes could redefine their social class status in a world where consumer goods were becoming more affordable to the masses.[14] Pierre Bourdieu also considers the links between social class and the practices of consumption but argues that wealth is not enough to define social class status. He uses the concept of cultural capital to explain the ways in which higher levels of education and social etiquette are used by the middle and upper classes to differentiate and reject 'popular' or obvious forms of consumption.[15]

Alcohol consumption must also be considered within the context of the expanding capitalist system. Jean Baudrillard considers the question of how needs for commodities are generated and argues that needs are not somehow 'magically' present within consumer objects.[16] Instead, the practices of marketing and advertising go further than creating the need to buy specific objects to create the need to buy almost any object.[17] In order to circumvent temperance ideology and reach consumers, alcohol producers had to invent reasons to buy alcohol and promote drinking as a desirable activity that symbolised cultural ideals. Michel de Certeau goes further to argue that consumers actively produce rather than consume meanings in objects.[18] De Certeau is concerned with ordinary people's engagement with consumption which he believes operates in a way that circumvents and subverts the dominant social order.[19] Building on Michel Foucault's concepts of power and discipline, he proposes that within the grid of discipline that exists to maintain the dominant social order, the 'consumer grid' operates as both a means of social control and political resistance.[20] In terms of alcohol consumption the relationship between drinkers and drinks may be guided by dominant social and cultural norms and values. However, the act of drinking creates a space that holds power for consumers and thus has meaning. The idea of a consumer grid allows agency for consumers to engage with alcohol in different ways for different reasons—sometimes challenging or resisting dominant cultural values.

This book engages with a range of perspectives in order to provide an analysis of alcohol production and consumption between 1872 and 1914. The problems of alcohol were evident during this time but there is another side to the story of drinking in late Victorian and Edwardian Britain. The book is thematically divided into three Parts which deal with different aspects of alcohol production and consumption. Part I explores the ways in which alcohol consumers were imagined and represented in political discourse. Chapter 2 considers the complexities of the drink question in the nineteenth century with an overview of the political responses to the issues of alcohol sale and consumption which resulted in stricter licensing laws later in the century. It then examines the impact this legislation had on alcohol producers and retailers who formed local and national trade defence organisations. One of the ways to promote and protect business interests was through the publication of weekly or monthly trade journals. The main purpose of these journals was to harness interest and support in trade defence activities and to promote and advertise local and national businesses. The chapter examines the ways in which the drink trade endeavoured to 'reinvent' their business as a respectable and vital part of British society. Chapter 3 investigates ideas about the 'great army of drinkers' that continued to drink alcohol despite moral pressure and political control of alcohol sale and consumption. One of the richest sources of information on alcohol consumers lies within the reports of parliamentary enquiries on alcohol held during the second half of the nineteenth century. During these enquiries, witnesses from across Britain gave detailed accounts of drinking within their towns, cities and districts. This provides insights into different types of drinking behaviour and also into the ways in which alcohol consumers were imagined and portrayed.

Chapter 4 continues the analysis of alcohol consumers but shifts the focus on to women drinkers. If men can be defined as a 'great army' of drinkers then women were the 'secret army' whose drinking behaviour was often shrouded by the constraints of gender norms and values or encased in ideas about deviancy and immorality. The chapter considers the division between women's public and private drinking and shows that women's drinking behaviour challenged patriarchal control and the ideals of femininity. Chapter 5 examines the issues that surrounded the types of alcoholic drinks sold to the public. It was widely believed that the types and qualities of alcohol sold and consumed within pubs and other drinking places influenced drinking behaviour. The quality of beer, wine and spirits varied enormously and some brewers and publicans used adulterants to enhance the quality, taste or strength of the liquor sold. Strong alcoholic drinks and those adulterated with other intoxicants were believed to have adverse effects on the behaviour of alcohol consumers.

Part II has three case studies of the nineteenth century drink trade. Chapter 6 considers the tactics of the brewing industry by focusing on one of the largest and most successful brewers in Britain, Bass & Co. Ltd. In order to compete in a growing domestic and foreign market for beer, Bass began to use advertising as a means of reaching larger groups of consumers. By appealing to notions of Britishness and Empire, Bass secured a market for their products and established a strong brand image. The company also used ideas about the supposed health giving properties of beer in order to boost dwindling sales towards the end of the century. Chapter 7 examines the motives of distillers with case studies of two whisky producers, Buchanan and Walker who successfully cultivated a market for Scotch whisky in England. James Buchanan ensured that his company's brands of blended whisky were conspicuously consumed by the British elites through the contract to supply to the Houses of Parliament and by securing Royal warrants. Chapter 8 considers the alcohol retail trade with a case study of one of the leading wine and spirit merchants in the Victorian period, W & A Gilbey, which restructured its business model due to pressure from customers to supply branded products. In the late Victorian period, particular brands of wine, champagne and spirits became more popular because they were associated with ideas about quality and taste. The company realised that in an emerging consumer culture, the power or 'illusion' of the brand held great commercial profit.

Part III considers the way in which alcohol was used and the different drinking cultures that emerged in the Victorian and Edwardian periods. Chapter 9 considers the use of alcohol by the medical profession in the last quarter of the nineteenth century. This was a time when doctors began to debate the efficacy of alcohol as a therapeutic drug and the moral implications of prescribing alcohol to patients. Alcohol was still used to treat a wide range of psychological and physiological illnesses but debates existed over the issue of therapeutic nihilism—whether alcohol did more harm than good and while some doctors held faith in its therapeutic qualities, others disagreed. An analysis of hospital records which show that alcohol use gradually declined in the period leading up to the First World War when the financial and moral cost of alcohol began to impact upon its popularity as a prescribed medicine. Chapter 10 examines the practice of drinking alcohol for health reasons. This was driven in part by the use of alcohol in medical practice but also by commercial factors, which played a significant role in promoting ideas about the health giving benefits of consuming certain alcoholic drinks. The chapter explores the ideas and controversies that surrounded the medicinal use of alcohol through a case study of Wincarnis Tonic Wine, which was one of the leading brands of tonic wine in the late nineteenth century. Political and medical debates existed about the therapeutic value of proprietary tonic wines which were sold and purchased as a means of self-medication for a range of psychological and physiological ailments.

Chapter 11 explores the drinking cultures of the working classes through analysis of oral history interviews conducted in the 1970s on surviving Victorians and Edwardians. These interviews reveal another side to working class drinking, where alcohol consumption revolved around family life, work and leisure. This stands in contrast to the way in which working class drinking was often portrayed as either 'carnivalesque' or 'teetotal' in political discourse. In fact, everyday working class drinking was much more humdrum and routine. In contrast, Chapter 12 considers drinking cultures of the middle and upper classes where there was a desire to consume alcohol in a conspicuous manner in order to reflect and promote social status. One of the key ways of achieving this was to consume the 'right' sorts of drinks in the 'right' kind of places. The chapter considers the way that men and women consumed alcohol within private spaces: in the home and within gentlemen's clubs. The domestic context of alcohol consumption was governed by rules of social etiquette, which both demonstrated and reinforced social class and gender values. The chapter provides a case study of alcohol consumption within two of London's top gentlemen's clubs: The Athenaeum and The Reform Club. The wine committees within gentlemen's clubs were tasked with cultivating and upholding particular standards of taste in alcoholic drinks. The men who drank in the clubs had the freedom and finances that allowed them to do so and therefore they expected to be served only the finest quality alcoholic drinks. As guardians of taste, the wine committees ensured that the alcohol consumed in gentlemen's clubs reflected the class and gender status of club members.

NOTES

1. Harrison B. 1971. *Drink and the Victorians: The Temperance Question in England 1815–1872*: London: Faber & Faber.
2. Weir R. B. 1984. 'Obsessed with Moderation: The Drink Trades and the Drink Question 1870–1930': *British Journal of Addiction*: Volume 79: pp. 93–107.
3. May C. 1997. 'Habitual Drunkards and the Invention of Alcoholism 1800–1850': *Addiction Research*: Volume 5:2.
4. Greenaway J. 2003. *Drink and British Politics Since 1830: A Study in Policy Making*: Basingstoke: Palgrave MacMillan.
5. Gutzke D. 1989. *Protecting the Pub: Brewers and Publicans Against Temperance*: Suffolk: The Boydell Press; Weir R. B. 1984. 'Obsessed with Moderation'.
6. Nicholls J. 2011. *The Politics of Alcohol: A History of the Drink Question in England*: Manchester: Manchester University Press.
7. Berridge V. 2013. *Demons: Our Changing Attitudes to Alcohol, Tobacco and Drugs*. Oxford: Oxford University Press.
8. Berridge V. 2013: location 1673.
9. Briggs A. 1985. *Wine For Sale: Victoria Wine and the Liquor Trade 1860–1984*: London: B.T. Batsford Ltd.
10. Duis P. 1998. *The Saloon: Public Drinking in Chicago and Boston, 1880–1920*: Chicago: University of Illinois Press; Powers M. 1998. *Faces Along the Bar: Lore and Order in the Workingmen's Saloon, 1870–1920*: Chicago: University of Chicago Press; Dikotter F., Laarmann L., and Xun Z. 2004. *Narcotic Culture: A History of Drugs in China*: Chicago, Chicago University Press; Zheng Y. 2005. *The Social Life of Opium in China*: Cambridge: Cambridge University Press; Heron C. 2003. *Booze: A Distilled History*: Toronto: Between The Lines; Gately I. 2009. *Drink: A Cultural History of Alcohol*: New York: Gotham Books.
11. Mitchell T. 2004. *Intoxicated Identities: Alcohol Power in Mexican History and Culture*: London: Routledge: p. 6.
12. Klein R. 1993. *Cigarettes Are Sublime*: London: Duke University Press.
13. Klein R. 1993: p. 2.
14. Veblen T. 1889/1994. *The Theory of the Leisure Class*: New York: Dover Publications Inc.
15. Bourdieu P. 1984/2010. *Distinction: A Social Critique of the Judgment of Taste*: London: Routledge.
16. Baudrillard J. 2003. 'The Ideological Genesis of Needs', in (eds.) Clarke D. B., Doel M., and Housiaux K. *The Consumption Reader*: London: Routledge: pp. 255–259.
17. Baudrillard J. 2003: p. 256.

18. de Certeau M. 2003. 'The Practice of Everyday Life', in (eds.) Clarke D. B., Doel M., and Housiaux K. *The Consumption Reader.* London: Routledge: pp. 259–267.
19. de Certeau M. 2003: p. 259.
20. de Certeau M. 2003: p. 260.

PART I

Drinkers

This part contains four chapters that consider the way that Victorian alcohol consumers were imagined and represented in political discourse. The chapters draw upon the rich, qualitative and quantitative data found in the various parliamentary enquiries on alcohol that took place in the second half of the nineteenth century. At these enquiries, expert witnesses offered testimonies and opinions on the causes and consequences of alcohol consumption, often revealing the fears and prejudices that surrounded issues of drunkenness. Yet the witnesses also described the many different types of drinking behaviour that ranged across social class, gender, occupation, ethnicity and regional location.

CHAPTER 2

The Spectre of the Drunkard

The issue of drunkenness cast a long shadow over the Victorian period and effectively masked ideas about the social benefits or pleasures to be gained from alcohol consumption. Ideas about the drunkard fuelled political and moral debates about the extent of liquor controls in Britain and drunkenness was the bane of the drink trade; leading to political organisation and the formation of trade defence leagues later in the period. As ideas about the causes and extent of drunkenness changed, so too did the proposed solutions and in the last quarter of the nineteenth century, the parliamentary enquiries came thick and fast as the drink question topped political agendas.

This chapter provides an overview of the political responses to the issues of drunkenness in the Victorian period. The common enemy of both the state and the drink trade was the drunkard—a figure that emerged from public fears and moral concern about the drinking culture of the urban working classes which was constantly on public show—spilling onto the streets of industrial cities and towns, threatening public order and obstructing social and moral progress. By the late nineteenth century, the drunkard was believed to dwell not only on city streets, prisons and workhouses but also in asylums and hospitals. Although thought to exist mainly among the labouring population, the drunkard did not respect other social boundaries and breached gender, region, age, religion and ethnicity. The drunkard was viewed as a social pest and a danger to civilised and progressive society but perhaps most notably, the drunkard posed a very real threat to the majority of moderate drinkers

© The Author(s) 2018
T. Hands, *Drinking in Victorian and Edwardian Britain*,
https://doi.org/10.1007/978-3-319-92964-4_2

13

because the political measures taken to thwart intemperance affected everyone. Towards the end of the century, as the grip of tighter licensing laws took hold, the drink trade made efforts to legitimise their existence as a vital and respectable part of British society.

THE LEGISLATIVE JIGSAW

The 1899 Report of the Royal Commission on Liquor Licensing Laws contained a summary of the various parliamentary commissions on alcohol held during the nineteenth century.[1] The summary report was commissioned by Lord Peel (1829–1912) who chaired the enquiry for most of its duration from 1897 to 1899. David Fahey notes that Peel's appointment was mainly due to his reputation for impartiality but during the course of the enquiry, for some unknown reason, he underwent 'a drastic conversion to temperance principles.'[2] Peel's conversion split the committee who then produced two reports that differed over their recommendations for reducing the numbers of public houses and granting compensation for loss of licenses. By the end of the nineteenth century, the drink question must have seemed like a legislative jigsaw puzzle composed of a succession of ill-fitting political strategies. Peel perhaps regarded it as his task to make a decisive impact upon the confusion of liquor licensing and in order to do so, he enlisted the skills of Mr R. A. Smith, an archaeologist at the British Museum. Exactly why he chose an archaeologist for this job is unclear. However, Smith's task was to review the various parliamentary enquiries on alcohol sale, licensing and intemperance which spanned the course of the century.

Smith's survey began in 1817 with the Select committee on the State of Metropolitan Police and the Licensing of Victuallers and ended in 1888 with the Select Committee on Sunday Closing Acts. During that time, there were 28 parliamentary enquiries into the issues surrounding alcohol sale and consumption in England, Wales, Scotland and Northern Ireland.[3] Each major enquiry was subjected to a meticulous analysis, which formed part of a concise overview of the political process relating to alcohol throughout most of the nineteenth century. The report showed that by the end of the century, intemperance remained a pressing political issue despite numerous enquiries and legislative attempts to control the drink trade and limit alcohol consumption. Yet Peel did not believe that this marked any kind of failure in the political process. On the contrary, he believed that Smith's report highlighted the important work done by parliamentary enquires

> It is commonly asserted that such enquiries never result in anything. Anyone at all familiar with the liquor laws and their history, who will glance at these pages, will see how wide of the truth these assertions are; even from the point of view of those who regard immediate legislation as the only test, and forget the work done, sometimes constructive, sometimes beneficially destructive, in the formation and education of opinion.[4]

Peel had faith in the political process and the summary report was perhaps intended as a testament to the complexity and thoroughness of the parliamentary investigations into the issues that surrounded the sale and consumption of alcohol. From a historical perspective, Smith's report is not only useful in providing a concise chronological summary of the main parliamentary enquiries but also as a means of identifying and situating the issues that surrounded the drink question and the various solutions proposed over the course of the century (see Appendix for the full table of enquiries).

The report began in 1818 when it was felt that the major brewers held a monopoly of tied (brewery owned) public houses in England and Wales and as a consequence, the public were forced to buy poor quality, over-priced beer and spirits. The solution was The 1830 Beer Act which was intended to weaken the position of the major brewers, discourage spirit drinking and promote the sale and consumption of better quality beer. However, this was a tall order considering the tempting and plentiful supply of cheap beer and spirits available to the burgeoning working classes within industrial towns and cities. The failure of the Beer Act to tackle intemperance was a constant theme during The 1834 Select Committee on Intoxication Among the Labouring Classes. It was believed that working-class drunkenness was the result of ingrained and problematic drinking customs; this belief essentially placed excessive drinking as a central feature of working-class life. The Beer Act was thought to have exacerbated drunkenness because it led to the proliferation of pubs and cheaper drinks. Therefore, the solutions proposed by the 1834 Committee were to limit access to alcohol by reducing pub numbers, regulating licensing and promoting alternative drinks such as tea and coffee. These were fairly radical recommendations for the time as they ran counter to laissez-faire principles and the rights of 'free men' to drink whatever and whenever they chose. However, the recommendations were, in Peel's opinion at least, the result of a thorough investigation of the drink problem, which he believed some of the later committees had failed to achieve. The parliamentary committees of the 1850s and 1860s had to deal with different aspects of the drink question and if their investigations and recommendations appeared weak to Peel, it was perhaps because they were in a sense dealing with a new set of problems that came in the wake of The 1830 Beer Act.

By mid-century, it was no longer a case of blaming drunkenness on the customs of the working classes or on the practices of brewers. Instead, drunkenness was explicitly linked to increases in poverty, crime and disorder among the working classes. Industrialisation and urbanisation had created new drinking cultures, and the Beer Act was instrumental in this process. It was believed that since the 1830s, there were more pubs of poorer quality and more 'bad characters' drinking than ever before.[5] The Beer Act had forged a distinction between beerhouses and pubs selling beer and spirits, which in turn fuelled competition to sell even more cheap spirits and beer to working-class populations. The solutions proposed were to tighten and simplify the licensing system and to also promote counter attractions for the working classes to steer them away from drunkenness and point them towards the sober pastimes offered by rational recreation.

The mid-century climate of moral improvement was evident in the 1850s and 1860s parliamentary commissions that examined the licensing system. By this time, the temperance movement was at its peak and drunkenness was encased within a moral framework but this was a framework still supported by laissez-faire ideology which favoured freedom of commerce. In effect, people had the absolute right to sell and consume alcohol but getting drunk was viewed as an individual moral failing. The type of alcohol consumed by the industrial working classes was also a cause of concern and spirit drinking in particular was singled out as a pernicious cause of intemperance. Therefore, one of the aims of The 1860 Wine and Refreshment Houses Act was to promote the sale and consumption of wine, which was not only less intoxicating than spirits but was also believed to promote more 'civilised' drinking habits.

However, by the 1870s drunkenness among the urban working classes was thought to prevail and it was no longer just a moral failing or a cause of crime and poverty but it was also believed to cause physical and mental illness.[6] With the weight of this added problem, the drink question sank beneath the buoyancy of laissez faire. At a political level there was a pressing need to reform the licensing system, rein in the power of the drink trade and 'rescue' the working classes from the moral and physical ravages of intemperance. As Harrison notes, The 1872 Licensing Act may have marked a minor victory for the temperance movement but it did not erase the issue of intemperance, which carried on regardless until the tighter licensing restrictions brought in during the First World War.[7] However, the parliamentary enquiries after 1872 were no longer constrained to the same extent by laissez faire—the state had already taken its first major step towards tighter control of alcohol sale and consumption. The main question driving the parliamentary enquiries after 1872 was the extent to which those controls should impinge upon the rights to sell and consume alcohol.

By the time that Peel chaired the 1897 commission, there was a vast array of proposed reforms to the licensing system ranging across a spectrum of direct state control of the alcohol trade to stepping up local powers to control licensing. As James Nicholls notes, the sheer number of proposed schemes was staggering but it was indicative of the general push towards restricting the trade in alcohol.[8] The drunkard had not exactly disappeared but was instead reimagined as the undesirable and often detestable product of a morally questionable profit-driven industry. Therefore, increasingly, the drink trade fell under the spotlight of public and political scrutiny for its culpability in creating the social problems associated with drunkenness. This was evident in another parliamentary enquiry held at the end of the century. In 1895 The Departmental Committee on Habitual Offenders (Scotland) dealt extensively with issues related to drunkenness in towns and cities across Scotland. Police statistics showed higher levels of drink-related crime in Scotland as compared to England and one of the committee's tasks was to investigate the causes of drink-related crime. There was the suggestion that policing tactics varied, and that in England, the lower number of arrests could be due to more lax procedures for dealing with drunkenness.[9] However some witnesses pointed the finger of blame towards publicans who continued to supply alcohol to drunken people

There are some publicans—perhaps we can hardly say a majority or minority—who are very conscientious but there are others that are not so. There is no doubt that publicans know drunkards who go in and get drunk week after week. They are known to the police, to their neighbours, and to the publicans to be drunkards and yet they are supplied in these houses till they are drunk.[10]

Throughout that enquiry, Scottish publicans constantly came under scrutiny as a potential source of drink-related crime and public disorder. Scotland seemed to have a more widespread problem with drunkenness and the drink trade was held to account. It therefore became necessary for the trade to mount a defence against further political and legislative 'attacks' and promote its business as both vital and respectable. Above all it had to distance itself from the drunkard.

THE PROBLEMS OF PROMOTING
A 'HAPPINESS INDUCING BUSINESS'

In the late Victorian period, Scottish alcohol producers and retailers formed local and national trade defence organisations. One of the ways to promote and protect business interests was through the publication of weekly or monthly trade journals. In Scotland three of the prominent trade journals were *The Scottish Wine, Beer and Spirits Trades Review*, *The Victualing Trades Review* and *The National Guardian*, all of which circulated from around the 1880s onwards. The main purpose of these journals was to harness interest and support in trade defence activities and to promote and advertise local and national businesses. The journals also reported on national drink issues such as parliamentary enquiries on alcohol, legislation and temperance campaigning. What really stands out from the journals is the absolute conviction that the drink trade was unfairly targeted because it was a legitimate and respectable business which served the public and generated substantial revenue for the nation. There was however no escaping the fact that it was a business that dealt in the somewhat controversial realm of intoxication. An article on 'why people drink' in *The National Guardian* in 1913 described the act of consuming alcohol as 'a happiness inducing business' and this in essence captures the way the drink trade aimed to be perceived both internally and externally.[11]

One of the themes that arose constantly within the journals was the allegedly 'ludicrous' and 'fanatical' standpoint of the temperance movement, particularly the teetotal faction. Articles that reported on temperance meetings or rallies did so with a mercilessly scathing and hostile tone. An article on the Scottish temperance societies in *The National Guardian* in 1904 launched an attack on the perceived failings of the temperance movement. After sixty years of campaigning, drunkenness prevailed and it was felt that the movement had achieved little more than to 'denounce the publican and pass the drunkard by.'[12] The 1902 Licensing Act had, of course, ramped up the restrictive nature of alcohol sale and control. Most importantly, the act put the onus on publicans and retailers to control the sale of drink and stem drunkenness within their establishments. It was felt that this singled out publicans as the purveyors of social evils

> Outside of fanaticism, every-one knows that licenses in the hands of respectable men, who respect the law and are respected by it, are legitimate and necessary, and their holding a respectable and necessary vocation.[13]

The counter-argument to the teetotal view was that the sale of drink was a legitimate and necessary vocation and a respectable one at that. The trade journals were therefore driven to promote and advertise the positive side of the liquor trade. An article in *The Scottish Wine, Beer and Spirits Trades Review* in 1895 reported on the annual festival of the Glasgow Wine, Beer and Spirits Trades Employees Benevolent Association. The main speech, given by Mr George MacLauchlan, the Vice President of the Association, focused on the 'slander of temperance extremists'

> A Trade the capital embarked in which exceeds 2 million Sterling; a Trade contributing to the revenue of the country to an extent of 40 million; a Trade funding employment for about 2 million of our population cannot be ignored and which commands imperative public recognition. What other trade in Glasgow contributes to any such extent? None ... It is with sobriety, education and intelligence that out Trade prospers and can only prosper. The curse of our Trade is the drunkard, the friend - the sober (applause). I admit there are men so constituted that they cannot, without serious consequences, taste alcohol at all. These are the small and numerically trifling exception, although it is the example furnished by them that is seized upon by our opponents as warranting an attack upon our Trade thereby falsifying alike logic and reason.[14]

MacLauchlan gave a rousing speech which delivered a strong argument and raised some key questions· if the local and national economy benefitted from the sale of alcohol, why the lack of gratitude? And if the majority of consumers drank in a moderate and respectable fashion, why attribute drunkenness to the liquor trade? Surely that was evidence enough that the trade served the public in a responsible way. Yet the one damning thing that made all that irrelevant was the very thing that kept the liquor trade afloat: alcohol. There simply was no way to guarantee that an intoxicant that came in so many varieties and strengths could *always* be consumed in a moderate and respectable fashion—the spectre of the drunkard was proof of that.

It was also difficult for 'respectable' members of the liquor trade to avoid the shadow cast by the disreputable side of the business. Therefore, many articles in the trade journals, particularly after 1900, dealt with the issues of unlicensed shebeens and bogus drinking clubs. One article in *The Victualing Trades Review* in 1904 offered an expose on a bogus club in Glasgow's East End. It claimed that there were around 200 bogus drinking clubs operating in Glasgow and that most sold cheap 'raw' whisky and poor quality beer. The clubs opened after the pubs closed on Saturdays and Sundays and remained open until the small hours of the morning. The article reported on a club known as The Literary and Social Institution in which it claimed there was:

> ... no literature, and the social intercourse of the members lay princi-
> pally in discussions as to what would win the 'back-end' handicap at
> Newmarket, forthcoming prize fights and the like. If heavy drinking
> counts as social intercourse, then the club really fulfilled to the hilt one of
> its missions for I have seen more liquor put away here in a couple of hours
> than would be sold over the bar in a small public house in a day.[15]

As a consequence of increasingly restrictive licensing and forced reductions in pub numbers, the trade knew that in order to survive, it had to be seen to operate in a respectable manner. It was therefore important to differentiate and distance themselves from disreputable vendors and drunken customers. Another article in *The National Guardian* in 1908 explored the issue of publicans and intemperance

> The publican alone, among merchants, habitually refuses undesirable busi-
> ness and he necessarily regards his drunken customer with aversion. He
> does not wish such to enter his shop ... respectable people will not fre-
> quent a bar patronized by the vicious and disorderly and in order to keep

his respectable customers pleased and content, the proprietor discourages traffic with obnoxious characters.[16]

A well-run establishment serving respectable, moderate-drinking customers was the trade ideal and this was precisely the image that publicans and licensed victuallers endeavoured to cultivate and promote both publicly and within their own ranks. Still, there was no escaping the 'threat' of drunkenness posed by the substance they dealt in. So, it was also important that alcohol itself was regarded not as a dangerous intoxicant but rather as a benign social lubricant. The trade journals carried many articles that promoted the social side of drinking by reporting on different pubs, drinking occasions and drinking customs in different countries. A piece in *The Victualling Trades Review* from 1900 listed the 'drinks of great men' and included Otto von Bismarck the German Chancellor who, as a 'staunch patriot' was known to drink mainly German beer and German wine. Gladstone drank claret and port and used a mix of sherry and egg yolk as a 'vocal lubricant' before public speaking, and Balfour preferred port.[17] The light-hearted tone of the piece did not disguise its intent to promote alcohol consumption as an intrinsic attribute found among 'great men'. There were few teetotallers listed and much use was made of the term 'moderate drinking'.

A constant theme throughout the years leading up to 1914 was the issue of why people consumed alcohol at all and it was vital that the trade devised reasons for drinking other than getting drunk. This was particularly the case in Scotland with the passing of The Temperance (Scotland) Act in 1913, which gave local voters the right to withhold licenses to sell alcohol in their districts. The looming threat of local veto meant that there had to be good reasons for drinking alcohol. An article in *The National Guardian* in 1913 written by 'a medical man' explored the psychological effects of alcohol

What the vast majority of persons who drink alcohol drink do it for is not because they like the taste of it, nor because they are thirsty, but for what is sometimes called its physiological effect, but what ought to be called its psychological effect—that is to say, in plain terms, because it makes them feel jolly. It raises their spirits. It confers happiness. It gives them a good conceit of themselves. Is it any wonder that it is so much valued by the English, who are so wanting in this useful sentiment? ... if it is taken regularly and always with the same moderation, although the full euphoric effect is not produced, some effect is produced; and the regular imbiber of moderate doses of alcohol is so much better off than the abstainer that though he does not attain the hilarious exhilaration of his first dose, he yet reaches a placid contentment, a good natured geniality.[18]

It was important for the trade to identify and promote the positive aspects of alcohol consumption. These could be social uses in dining and conviviality or drinking healths and toasts. Or as this quote demonstrates, alcohol could have the psychological effect of 'lifting the spirits' or making people 'feel jolly.' However, the key to securing the continued fortunes of the trade in alcohol lay in the direction of moderate drinking. This was known to the trade and also to alcohol consumers, as demonstrated by the formation of The National Temperate Society in Manchester in 1907. The society was formed to 'combat the uncalled for interference with the liberties of citizens who choose to indulge to a moderate extent in alcoholic liquors.'[19] *The Manchester Courier* reported on the activities of the society, which by 1907 had 700 members who embarked on 'missionary work' in local pubs to try and induce customers to form branches

That class of the community known as 'moderate drinkers', men who after a day's work enjoy an hour or two's social intercourse on licensed premises, have discovered that their rights were being menaced, and in one part of Manchester have banded themselves together under the title of The National Temperate Society with the object of resisting any unreasonable interference with the liberty of pleasing themselves.[20]

In the shadow cast by the spectre of the drunkard, drink became a political issue and by the turn of the century, the principles of laissez faire no longer supported an industry that dealt in intoxication. Increased state control over alcohol sale and consumption impacted not only upon the livelihoods and reputation of the drink trade but also on alcohol consumers and as the quote above demonstrates, some were prepared to campaign for the freedom to drink. The members of the National Temperate Society argued that not all paths led to Rome—in other words, not every drinker was a drunkard. There were many reasons why people across Britain consumed alcohol and many different types of drinking behaviour, other than drunkenness.

NOTES

1. House of Commons Parliamentary Papers (HCPP). 1899: c. 9076: Royal Commission on Liquor Licensing Laws: Volume XI: Précis of Minutes of Evidence: Appendix 5: Summary reports from Royal, Select and Departmental Committees on the liquor traffic in Great Britain and Ireland.
2. Fahey D. 1971. 'Temperance and the Liberal Party—Lord Peel's Report, 1899': *Journal of British Studies*: Volume 10:2: p. 135.
3. HCPP. 1899: c. 9076: Royal Commission on Liquor Licensing Laws: Volume XI: Précis of Minutes of Evidence: Appendix 5.
4. HCPP. 1899: c. 9076: Royal Commission on Liquor Licensing Laws: Volume XI: Précis of Minutes of Evidence: Appendix 5.
5. HCPP. 1899: c. 9076: Royal Commission on Liquor Licensing Laws: Volume XI: Précis of Minutes of Evidence: Appendix 5.
6. HCPP. 1899: c. 9076: Royal Commission on Liquor Licensing Laws: Volume XI: Précis of Minutes of Evidence: Appendix 5.
7. Harrison B. 1971. *Drink and the Victorians: The Temperance Question in England 1815–1872*: London: Faber & Faber: p. 12.
8. Nicholls J. 2011. *The Politics of Alcohol: A History of the Drink Question in England*: Manchester: Manchester University Press: pp. 130–131.
9. HCCP. 1897. The Departmental Commission on Habitual Offenders (Scotland): p. vi.
10. HCCP. 1897. The Departmental Commission on Habitual Offenders (Scotland): Testimony of Father John McMillan: p. 74.
11. 'Why Do People Take Alcohol?' *The National Guardian*: January 1913.
12. 'Why Do People Take Alcohol?' *The National Guardian*: January 1913.
13. 'Why Do People Take Alcohol?' *The National Guardian*: January 1913.
14. 'Wine, Spirits and Beer Trades Employees Festival': *The Scottish Wine, Spirit and Beer Trades Review*: 1895.
15. 'Sunday in a Drinking Club: The Unlicensed Pub': *The Victualing Trades Review*: 1904.
16. 'Publicans and Intemperance': *The National Guardian*: April 1908.
17. 'The Drinks of Great Men': *The Victualing Trades Review*: 1900.
18. 'Drunkenness and the Physiological Effect of Alcohol': *The National Guardian*: January 1913.
19. 'Moderate Drinkers: To Combat Teetotal Intolerance': *The Manchester Courier and Lancashire General Advertiser*: 11 April 1907.
20. 'Moderate Drinkers: To Combat Teetotal Intolerance': *The Manchester Courier and Lancashire General Advertiser*: 11 April 1907.

CHAPTER 3

The Great Army of Drinkers

There can be no doubt that the great majority of those who purchase and consume liquor are not guilty of intoxication, nor are the places where it is sold by any means so universally the scenes of drunkenness and disorder as to call for their universal suppression on that ground alone. It does not seem therefore either just or expedient that the perfectly moderate and harmless purchase and use of liquor by the majority of persons should be prevented because there are some who abuse the purchase and use of it to their own hurt and that of others.[1]

The Licensing Acts of 1869 and 1872 marked a turning point in British alcohol history. Laissez-faire policies were to some extent set aside because a greater degree of state control was considered necessary to prevent drunkenness and public disorder. Yet as the quote above shows, it was the nature and extent of alcohol controls that fuelled political debates and parliamentary enquiries in the late nineteenth century. The quote comes from the report of The Select Committee on Intemperance, which was appointed in 1877 to review the effects of the restrictive measures imposed by the Licensing Acts. Although the committee heard evidence of drunkenness across towns and cities in Britain, it rejected calls from temperance campaigners for strict licensing restrictions or for outright prohibition. The committee believed there were no grounds for such extreme measures because the majority of people drank moderately. In an analysis of the political manoeuvres of temperance campaigners, James Nicholls states that 'standing between radical teetotallers and the

© The Author(s) 2018
T. Hands, *Drinking in Victorian and Edwardian Britain*,
https://doi.org/10.1007/978-3-319-92964-4_3

sober millennium was an enormous army of moderate drinkers for whom teetotal reclamation meant nothing.'[2] In other words, moral suasion and legislative controls did little to deter the majority of people from consuming alcohol. A great army of drinkers was a force to be reckoned with—not only for temperance campaigners and politicians but also for the drink trade. In a political battle between government and commerce over alcohol control, consumers were not mere pawns of war. Instead, they were the agents of victory for either side. Therefore, gaining knowledge of this army of drinkers held enormous political value.

This chapter examines the efforts made at a political level to investigate the majority of drinkers in the late Victorian period. One of the richest sources of information on alcohol consumers lies within the reports of various parliamentary enquiries on alcohol held during the second half of the nineteenth century. During these enquiries, witnesses from across Britain gave detailed accounts of drinking within their towns, cities and districts. A close reading of the minutes of evidence reveals that alcohol consumers were imagined and represented in different ways at different times, often reflecting the changing social and cultural context of alcohol sale and consumption. The chapter draws upon evidence from four major parliamentary enquiries on alcohol in the latter half of the nineteenth century: The 1853 Select Committee on Public Houses (1853 enquiry), which was appointed to investigate the regulation of drinking establishments created in the wake of The 1830 Beer Act; The 1872 Select Committee on Habitual Drunkards (1872 enquiry) which examined the existing laws on the control of drunkenness; The 1877 Select Committee on Intemperance (1877 enquiry) which was appointed to investigate the causes and extent of intemperance across Britain and The 1897 Royal Commission on Liquor Licensing (1897 enquiry) which examined the laws relating to the sale and consumption of alcohol. Another important enquiry on alcohol was The 1890 Select Committee on British and Foreign Spirits (1890 enquiry), which was appointed in the interests of public health to examine the system for the manufacture and sale of spirits.

These enquires provide rich sources of qualitative and quantitative information on alcohol consumers. This evidence must however be weighed against the political nature of the enquiries. The reports could to some extent be regarded as discourses of alcohol consumption, which provide a distorted 'top-down' account of alcohol consumers framed by political motives and moral concerns about intemperance. Yet it is important to consider that many committee members were themselves alcohol consumers and often the line of questioning reveals as much about their ideas as the evidence given by witnesses. A close reading of the minutes of evidence reveals insights into ideas about the majority of alcohol consumers—who they were, what they drank and where they drank and how ideas about moderate drinking and drunkenness changed over time. This chapter considers the extent to which these ideas about drinkers, drinks and drinking places shaped impressions of alcohol consumers.

'Is There Anything Among the Working Classes Like a Moderate Drinker'?

The parliamentary enquiries on alcohol in the last half of the nineteenth century largely focused on investigating issues of intemperance primarily but not exclusively among the working classes. During the 1877 enquiry, one of the committee members asked Joseph Chamberlain, then an MP for Birmingham 'We hear a great deal about moderate drinkers; is there anything among the working classes like a moderate drinker; that is to say, is there anything as a rule in the way of a medium between a teetotaller and a man going utterly into drink?'[3] In reply to the question, Chamberlain stated that in his opinion there were many cases of 'occasional drunkards' and that habitual drunkards were a small minority in any social class. Yet he went on to provide evidence from a study on Saturday night drinking in Birmingham conducted by The UK Alliance, a prominent temperance organisation. The study showed that on one Saturday night alone, 14,165 people came out of 35 pubs during the three hours of observation and that 838 of those were deemed drunk. Chamberlain argued that the study highlighted the weakness in police statistics which under-represented the extent of drunkenness in larger cities. He stated that the drunkenness observed on that Saturday night was 1500 times greater than the drunken arrests recorded on the same night.[4] It was perhaps Chamberlain's aim to present evidence of widespread drinking among the working classes and therefore it did not matter if the Saturday night pub goers in Birmingham were moderate drinkers or habitual drunkards. Nor did the fact that 14,165 people were drinking on a Saturday night yet only 838 were deemed drunk which meant that over 13,000 pub goers remained relatively sober. Temperance advocates recorded the numbers of what they believed to be drunk people leaving pubs. The committee cross-examined Chamberlain on the reliability of a study conducted by temperance campaigners who were unlikely to be impartial when classifying drunkenness. Just how they classified drunkenness is unclear but it is likely to have been along the lines of 'falling down drunk' and since most people leaving the pubs were not showing visible signs of falling-down drunkenness, it could have reasonably been argued that most drank moderately. Yet this appeared to be less important than the sheer numbers of drinkers.

The 1877 enquiry heard evidence from a range of witnesses from urban and rural regions of Britain who described different types of drinking and drunkenness. The Chief Constable of Newcastle-upon-Tyne, Captain Samuel James Nicholls gave evidence of drinking patterns in the Newcastle area. Nicholls described the character of the Newcastle population as manufacturing and industrial—chiefly mechanical engineering, shipbuilding, coal mining and the chemical industries. He noted that although Newcastle was a thriving industrial city, it was also prone to frequent trade depressions. Nicholls described the pattern of working men's drinking which centred on their working lives and hours of employment. He believed that drinking was more of a 'nuisance' at the weekend when men finished work at 1 p.m. on a Saturday then went to the pub and drank away their wages until closing time. The drinking continued on a Sunday evening and all-day Monday, as many men in Newcastle still observed the unofficial day-off work known as Saint Monday. Nicholls described how miners in the region around Newcastle would 'come into the moor' (which was a large section of common ground on the outskirts of Newcastle) on Saturdays for sporting events and then carry on to the local pubs in the evening. The miners would take part in rabbit coursing which Nicholls described as 'a very great nuisance to the respectable community, on account of the disgusting language used by competitors and their backers.'[5] Although Nicholls found the weekend leisure pursuits of Newcastle's miners somewhat distasteful, he linked their drinking habits to their type of employment. These were men employed in heavy industries and although many of them drank heavily at weekends, Nicholls believed that drunkenness was a problem mainly confined to poorer sections of the working classes and that the 'respectable classes' were becoming more sober. It is not clear from his evidence whether Nicholls' considered the miners to be 'respectable' but he did draw a distinction between heavy weekend drinking and the type of drunkenness that resulted in crime or public disorder.

The dichotomy thought to exist between the drinking habits of the 'respectable' and 'rough' working classes was also highlighted in the evidence given to the committee by a Preston magistrate Charles Roger Jackson. In the late nineteenth century, Preston was a manufacturing and mining town with a large Irish population. Jackson's evidence of the drinking habits of the working-class population mirrored that of Nicholls in that he believed most men drank at the weekends. The key difference was that the mill workers did not observe Saint Monday and therefore most drinking took place on the half-day Saturday holiday and Sunday evening. Jackson presented evidence from the Preston Savings Bank which detailed the employment status of depositors to make the point that not all men's wages were drunk away at the weekend. Most were mill workers, followed by plasterers, railwaymen, policemen, labourers, shopwomen, workwomen, milliners, book keepers, clerks, shopkeepers, tradesmen, farmers, gardeners, spinsters, widows and married women.[6] When asked for the point in presenting this evidence, Jackson replied that it was to show that money was being saved and not spent on drink and that not all of the working classes were frittering their wages away on drink every week but that some, arguably the more 'respectable' sections, were either abstaining or drinking moderately.

The witness testimonies of the 1877 enquiry showed that drinking was often an integral part of working men's lives, particularly in heavy industries, manufacturing and also in the armed services. The 1877 committee was keen to investigate the relationship that existed between working life and drinking habits in order to assess how the numbers of pubs and pub opening hours impacted upon the extent of intemperance. Some witnesses believed that working-class men drank away their wages at the weekend and that heavy drinking was the main reason for observing Saint Monday. However, there seemed to be a distinction drawn between heavy drinking and drunkenness and although both were considered problematic, some witnesses implied that the worst problems of drunkenness existed mainly among the lowest classes of society. In this sense, heavy weekend drinking and indeed drinking during working hours rested somewhere on a spectrum between moderate drinking and drunkenness. The witnesses seemed to acknowledge that heavy drinking was a part of working-class masculinity and therefore it was not viewed as particularly deviant or immoral—unless it led to or involved other 'social evils' such as gambling, domestic violence or prostitution. It appeared that some men drank heavily but still held down jobs and supported families. A sober industrial workforce may have been the moral and political ideal, but the 1877 enquiry was dealing with the realities of working-class life and it is clear that on a political level it was understood that working-class men's drinking habits varied.

It seemed to be difficult to pin down one definition or type of drunkenness. One witness at the 1877 enquiry, John Matthias Weylland of the London City Mission, reported on his observations of working-class drinking from visiting pubs, gin palaces and dram shops in London and from speaking with barmen, barwomen and customers. Weylland had previously given evidence before the 1853 enquiry on his observations of pubs in and around the Marylebone area of London. For the purposes of the 1877 enquiry, he revisited these pubs and noted any changes. Weylland claimed that there was a marked increase in spirit drinking among men and women, which he believed caused a 'great deal of drunkenness.'[7] When asked by the committee to define drunkenness, Weylland replied that he considered a man to be drunk when he had lost his reason and was not capable of receiving instruction. He believed that there was still a great deal of drinking among what he termed the 'roughs' or the 'drinking class' of London but that most 'other' working-class people were moderate drinkers.[8] Another witness, Major John Grieg who was the Chief Constable of Liverpool, was questioned about the extent of drunkenness in the city. He presented statistics which showed an overall increase in drunken arrests in the city from 11,439 in 1857 to 20,551 in 1876.[9] However, there were fluctuations in the numbers of arrests during this period. When asked to account for these fluctuations Grieg pointed towards the maritime population of Liverpool

> The floating population are, upon average, 20,000 seamen, increased by a west wind and decreased by an east wind. The docks are at our doors and the sailors come home, frequently with large arrears of pay to receive, which they spend thoughtlessly and most wickedly, I should say.[10]

Grieg argued that the west wind brought in more ships and sailors who had money to spend on leisure activities that mainly involved alcohol and prostitutes. The pubs, beer houses and brothels situated around the Liverpool docks area made their livelihoods from catering to the demands and desires of the maritime population. A west wind may have blown in more drunkenness but Grieg seemed aware that it was a transient and in some ways an inevitable consequence of Liverpool's status as

a major port. This perhaps required a more pragmatic approach to policing drunkenness. When cross-examined on the types of drunken arrests,
Grieg was asked to explain the category of 'semi-drunkenness' which
appeared in the police statistics. He defined 'semi drunkenness' as being
drunk but not sufficiently drunk to be locked up and explained that in
some cases, people were apprehended and taken to the station where
they would either sober up *en* route and go home or they would sober
up in the police station. In either case they would be released without
charge. This practice was not confined to Liverpool alone and witnesses
from other parts of Britain gave evidence of cases of 'simple' drunkenness that were not considered to be criminal and therefore not a matter
for the police. Indeed, Grieg stated that any officer who was found to
have locked up a person unnecessarily was dealt with 'severely'.[11] The
Chief Constable of Birmingham, Major Edwin Bond went further and
argued that legislation and over-policing of drunkenness could in fact
worsen the problem

> If instead of letting people have their natural refreshment in the way of
> their beer and their wine, we are constantly to be legislating upon the
> subject and damming it up into narrower limits, it will lead to very much
> worse troubles. I believe we should have secret drinking all round.[12]

Major Bond also believed that there was a difference between 'quietly
drunk' and 'drunk and disorderly' and when asked what measures were
taken by his constables to deal with a drunken man he stated that 'we do
not say anything to him if he does not say anything to anybody else.'[13]
Another witness at the 1877 enquiry, Superintendent George Turner of
the London Constabulary was asked to tell the committee what he called
'really drunk' and Turner replied

> There are so many degrees of drunkenness, that I can hardly define it; but
> if a man is staggering and he can go home, we let him go. I should say that
> man was drunk, but if he could walk straight and reasonable, I should say
> he was 'influenced' but not drunk.[14]

Turner was told reproachfully by the committee that he held 'a very high
standard of drunkenness.'[15] However this kind of pragmatic approach to
policing drunkenness perhaps saved police time and resources. The evidence from the police also highlights the difficulties that people had in

pinning down one universal definition of drunkenness. There was a sense that ideas about drunkenness varied regionally and that different constabularies had their own methods for dealing with drunkards. It seemed important to allow men to go about their business if they were not deemed to be a public nuisance. In a sense, this seemed to be protecting the rights of the majority of men to go out and have a drink without fear of being locked up.

This issue of police interference in drinking habits was, of course, part of the larger debate about the liberty to drink versus state control. Although the parliamentary committees were established primarily to investigate issues of intemperance, any legislation enacted would affect the majority of drinkers. It sometimes fell to committee members to represent the views of the majority of drinkers by cross-examining pro-temperance witnesses. One example of this was the question and answer exchange that occurred during the 1877 enquiry when the Reverend D Burns of The UK Alliance (a national temperance association) was questioned by the Bishop of Peterborough, William Magee, who held anti-temperance views.[16] When asked by Magee if he would interfere with the liberty of a man to drink alcohol in his own house, Burns replied that he would not. Magee seemed dissatisfied with this response and prodded him further

> *Magee*: You would not pass a law that he should only drink at certain hours in his own house?
> *Burns*: No.
> *Magee*: And you would not send a policeman to see whether he drank more than was good for him, or drank at improper hours?
> *Burns*: No.
> *Magee*: Why would you not do so; I presume the reason would be that you respect the liberty of the individual?
> *Burns*: Yes I would.
> *Magee*: You would prefer that he should be free in his own house than be sober?
> *Burns*: I should prefer him being both.
> *Magee*: Supposing that you could make or keep a man sober by sending a policeman in and preventing his drinking, you would not do so because that would be an interference with the liberty of the subject?
> *Burns*: It would be utterly impractical to do so.
> *Magee*: I am not asking whether it would be impracticable to do so, but would you do it?

Burns: I would not.

Magee: Therefore if the choice were between a man being drunk in his own house and being kept sober by a visit from a policeman, you would not send in your policeman to make him sober or keep him so; in other words being compelled to choose, in that case you would rather leave him free than force him to be sober; is that not so?

Burns: That would depend upon the circumstances. I do not think that you can lay down any broad principle to that effect. If the people of this country were so abusing this freedom of which your Lordship speaks, and they were systematically getting drunk in their own houses and thus destroying the State, I think measures of a very strong kind might be desirable; and even that interference with personal liberty might be desirable.

Magee: But there is no doubt that many persons do abuse their personal liberty at this moment by getting drunk; do you propose that all persons sober as well as drunken, shall be put under the restraint of a policeman, because of the conduct of these people in their own house?

Burns: Our Bill[17] does not propose to do that.

Magee: But your Bill does propose to deprive sober people of their drink, because of the abuse of drunken persons; do you propose to carry that out or not?

Burns: We propose only to interfere as far as the law has the right to interfere.[18]

This exchange highlights the extent to which ideas about the freedom to drink were grounded in the division between public and private drinking. One consequence of the reduced pub opening hours imposed by The 1869 and 1872 Licensing Acts, was the increased popularity of working men's clubs which were run by private members. These places were not regulated by the licensing acts and for this reason, private members clubs attracted the scorn of the drink trade and the wrath of temperance campaigners who viewed such establishments as stealing trade while promoting drunkenness among working men.[19] Throughout the 1877 and 1897 enquiries, witnesses were asked for their opinions or experiences of working men's clubs and whether they considered these to be genuine and beneficial or 'bogus' establishments that operated as unlicensed pubs. Views were mixed and some witnesses like Joseph Chamberlain argued that the working men's clubs in Birmingham were respectably run places that provided refreshments for men who worked late hours.[20] Others witnesses at the

1877 enquiry disagreed but the recommendations of the committee were that no change in the law regarding private clubs was deemed necessary.[21]

By 1897 the issue of working men's clubs lingered on. Witnesses such as Sir John Bridge, a senior London magistrate, argued that bogus clubs were a source of much illicit drinking.[22] However one of the committee members pointed out that the issue of private clubs was directed mainly at the working classes yet these clubs permeated the class system.[23] One witness at the 1897 enquiry was Algernon Bourke who the manager of Whites Club in London's West End. In the late nineteenth century, the London club scene was thriving and many gentlemen's clubs situated around Pall Mall and St James's were frequented by men in prominent positions such as the landed elites, politicians, businessmen and the intelligentsia. Bourke was asked if the London clubs generated substantial amounts of income from the sale of liquor. He replied that this was not the case and that clubs made most of their money from membership fees.[24] He claimed that although there was a large amount of alcohol sold within clubs, the prices charged were moderate because clubs did not pay any excise duties or license fees. He was then asked for his opinions on licensing private clubs and replied that a license would be unfair to the men who used the London clubs 'like a home' because this would restrict the hours of sale of alcohol. Bourke stated that in theory, Whites could sell liquor all day and night but in practice this did not happen and instead the club usually closed between 2 a.m. and 10 a.m. and any alcohol sold within these hours was by special arrangement only.[25] He was also asked if 'intoxication' had increased or decreased in the West End of London (the word drunkenness was never used) and replied that in his opinion there was a great decrease in drinking among the upper classes.

The issue of regulating private clubs was controversial because it was a further infringement upon the personal liberty of men to drink alcohol in private whenever they chose to do so. Working men's clubs and gentlemen's clubs were created through male alliances and as such they represented masculine spaces where men could escape from the public world to socialise and drink alcohol in private. In essence, all the men-only private clubs delivered the same social goals. Political and moral concerns about working-class drunkenness cast a shadow over the idea of working men's clubs. Yet it was never suggested that any of the London clubs could ever be 'bogus' and merely operate as unlicensed pubs and gambling dens. Implicit in the evidence about working men's and gentlemen's clubs was the assumption that 'genuine' clubs fostered moderate and respectable drinking habits. In a highly patriarchal culture, all men—including working-class men, had the right to socialise and drink in private. Even when the Licensing Act of 1902 made it compulsory for private clubs to be registered with local licensing authorities, this did not bring men's clubs into line with other licensed premises and therefore meant that to some extent, private drinking was still protected by law.

The issue of genuine and bogus private members clubs was one of many instances where the committee's sought to investigate the differences between respectably run and disreputable drinking places. During the 1897 enquiry, Sir John Bridge, a senior London Magistrate was asked if he could single out the worst types of pubs and beer shops. Bridge replied that he could not attach drunkenness to any particular drinking place, either licensed or illicit. However, another London magistrate, Alfred de Rutzen, believed that certain types of pubs encouraged more drunkenness. To illustrate his point, he gave an example of a London pub which by its design encouraged anonymous and sometimes illicit drinking

> I went down to see it and I saw this state of things, which rather astonished me. The particular bar or compartment in which this man had been served was shut off from the bar by high sides, and between the bar and the compartment was an erection of dark glass through which nobody could see, and the consequence was that the people who were being served in the compartment could not see over it, and the only way you could see under it was through a little opening which was exactly the height of a quart pot through which any drink might be handed out and the money taken. As a matter of fact, nobody could see any single person who was in the bar and therefore almost any offence might have been committed, such as serving children or serving a policeman, serving spirits to young people under 16, and almost every single offence of that sort could have been committed without any human being who was serving in the bar seeing anybody.[26]

Many late Victorian pubs were designed with compartments or separate bars that offered some degree of privacy for customers. For example, public bars sometimes contained compartments for the sale of liquor to be consumed off the premises and women sometimes drank in private closed-off bars.[27] Gin palaces, gin shops, vaults and dram shops were designed with less seating to attract high turnovers of customers, who drank quickly and left. Some witnesses regarded the profusion of pubs in cities and towns not as forming an integral and 'normal' part of daily life but rather as providing an escape from it.

A common theme running through the various parliamentary enquiries was that the working classes and particularly the poor were driven to drink through poor housing, poverty and a generally miserable existence. In the 1877 enquiry, John Bremner, a Manchester magistrate stated that in his opinion, the greatest numbers of pubs in Manchester were situated in the poorest areas with the worst types of housing.[28] Another witness at that enquiry, William Sproston Caine went further and argued that there was a direct link between the numbers of pubs and the death rates in certain areas of Liverpool.[29] Caine was a Liberal MP and fervent pro-temperance campaigner who held radical views on prohibition. He presented a map to the committee detailing the numbers of pubs and death rates in certain areas. When cross-examined by a somewhat sceptical sounding committee member who pointed out that death rates in poor areas may be linked to wider socio-economic factors, Caine stuck to his guns and argued that drinking, and particularly the trade in drink, caused death among the working classes.[30] The pro-temperance witnesses tended to give the most radical and in some cases, sensationalist accounts of the 'evils' of the drink trade. One witness, Alfred Eccles, a cotton mill owner from Salford, claimed that his village of White Coppice which in 1877 had no pubs or beer shops, was a prime example of the tragedies that could result from the trade in liquor. He stated that

> It is a singular fact that the people who have sold liquor in our district have been particularly liable to being burnt to death, and to accidents upon the railway and to having their children drowned etc. We had one beer seller who had his little child drowned within twelve months of his brother, who also kept a beer shop, having his child burnt to death; another brother was run over on the railway while in a state of intoxication and killed on the spot, and another beer shop keeper in our district had his little child drowned. The other beer shopkeeper committed suicide after being unsuccessful in two previous attempts at self-destruction.[31]

Given all this tragedy it was hardly surprising that White Coppice had no beer shops. Eccles held up his village as a model of temperance and sobriety but the committee seemed sceptical and asked if there was any shebeening (illegal drinking in unlicensed premises) in the village or if the locals went to nearby pubs in other villages. Eccles replied that there were no cases of shebeening and that he had 'never seen anyone' bring back beer from the nearest pub which was three quarters of a mile away.[32] One committee member then asked what people drank with their supper if they had no beer available locally. Eccles replied that they drank tea, water or milk.[33] He claimed that his village was a 'moral place' due to the absence of a pub and he could prove it because the local register of births showed no illegitimate conceptions. Yet the committee seemed to find it very difficult to believe that the people of White Coppice were entirely teetotal. Drinking table beer with dinner or supper was an integral part of the day for working-class people and there was a sense that the committee not only knew that but felt that working-class people were perhaps entitled to beer with their evening meal.

Other witnesses at the 1877 enquiry such as Professor Leoni Levi, a barrister and statistician, presented less moralistic evidence. Levi offered statistics to corroborate his theory that any increase in drunkenness was directly linked to an increase in trade which was a consequence of better wages among the working classes.[34] In this sense, the drink trade followed the money or vice versa and the result was intemperance. Some witnesses, and not just the pro-temperance ones seemed to find it hard to accept that the working classes even the more prosperous ones, went to pubs and other drinking places for reasons other than escapism or that the results of drinking were anything less than drunkenness. There was little discussion of the ways in which people drank for enjoyment and pleasure or to socialise or conduct business because the focus was always on intemperance and excess rather than on 'normal' or everyday drinking. For this reason, it was easier for some to view the drink trade as a 'great evil' that put profits before health, morality or social order. Ideas about municipal control of pubs, disinterested management schemes and counter-attractions for the working classes all stemmed from the belief that alcohol was something that the drink trade could not sell responsibly and the working classes could not consume moderately. Yet witnesses also gave evidence of a spectrum of working-class drinking that ranged from moderate consumption to 'falling down drunk'. Implicit in this type of evidence was the knowledge that not all working-class men were drunkards and that not all types of drinking were problematic and had to be policed. This highlights the larger debate that fuelled the drink question in the nineteenth century—that of the freedom to drink versus state control. Legislation that impacted upon men's rights to drink alcohol in public and in private had to be considered carefully since it was not only working-class men who were affected. Although this debate extended across class lines it did not cross the gender divide. Victorian society was highly patriarchal and, as the next chapter shows, this was reflected in attitudes towards all women's drinking behaviour, regardless of class status.

NOTES

1. House of Commons Parliamentary Papers (HCPP). 1878–1879: c. 113: 4th Report of The Select Committee of the House of Lords on Intemperance.
2. Nicholls J. 2011. *The Politics of Alcohol: A History of the Drink Question in England*: Manchester: Manchester University Press: p. 112.
3. HCPP. 1877: c. 171: First Report of the Select Committee of the House of Lords on Intemperance.
4. HCPP. 1877: c. 171: First Report of the Select Committee of the House of Lords on Intemperance: Evidence of Joseph Chamberlain.
5. HCPP. 1877: c. 271: Second Report of the Select Committee of the House of Lords on Intemperance: Evidence of Captain Nicholls.
6. HCPP. 1877: c. 271: Second Report of the Select Committee of the House of Lords on Intemperance: Evidence of Captain Nicholls.
7. HCPP. 1877: c. 418: Third Report from the Select Committee of the House of Lords on Intemperance: Evidence of John Matthias Weylland.
8. HCPP. 1877: c. 418: Evidence of John Matthias Weylland.
9. HCPP. 1877: c. 171: First Report from the Select Committee of the House of Lords on Intemperance: Evidence of Major John James Grieg, Chief Constable of Liverpool.
10. HCPP. 1877: c. 171: Evidence of Major John James Grieg.
11. HCPP. 1977. c. 171: First Report from the Select Committee of the House of Lords on Intemperance: Evidence of Major John James Grieg.
12. HCPP. 1877: c. 171: First Report from the Select Committee of the House of Lords on Intemperance: Evidence of Major Edwin Bond, Chief Constable of Birmingham.
13. HCPP. 1877: c. 171: First Report from the Select Committee of the House of Lords on Intemperance: Evidence of Major Edwin Bond, Chief Constable of Birmingham.
14. HCPP. 1877: c. 271: Second Report from the Select Committee of the House of Lords on Intemperance: Evidence of Superintendent George Turner, London Constabulary.
15. HCPP. 1877: c. 271: Evidence of Superintendent George Turner.
16. Brief biography of William Magee: https://en.wikisource.org/wiki/Magee,_William_Connor_%28DNB00%29: accessed 10/3/2016.

17. The bill that the Reverend referred to was The Permissive Bill submitted to parliament by Sir Wilfred Lawson in 1869. The Bill proposed that local ratepayers should be given power to decide on numbers of licensed premises within their districts.
18. HCPP. 1878: No. 338: Fourth Report of the Select Committee of the House of Lords on Intemperance: Evidence of Reverend D. Burns.
19. Gutzke D. 1989. *Protecting the Pub: Brewers and Publicans Against Temperance*: New Hampshire: The Boydell Press: pp. 192–194.
20. HCPP. 1877: c. 171: First Report of the Select Committee of the House of Lords on Intemperance: Evidence of Joseph Chamberlain.
21. HCPP. 1899: c. 9076: Royal Commission on Liquor Licensing Laws: Summary Report.
22. HCPP. 1897: c. 8355: First Report of the Royal Commission on Liquor Licensing Laws: Evidence of Sir John Bridge.
23. HCCP. 1897: c. 8355: Evidence of Sir John Bridge.
24. HCPP. 1877: c. 171: First Report of the Select Committee of the House of Lords on Intemperance: Evidence of Algernon Bourke.
25. HCPP. 1877: c. 171: First Report of the Select Committee of the House of Lords on Intemperance: Evidence of Algernon Bourke.
26. HCPP. 1897: c. 8355: First Report of the Royal Commission on Liquor Licensing Laws: Evidence of Albert de Rutzen.
27. Girourard M. 1990. *Victorian Pubs*. Unites States: Yale University Press: pp. 2–7.
28. HCPP. 1877: c. 171: First Report of the Select Committee of the House of Lords on Intemperance: Evidence of John Alexander Bremner.
29. HCPP. 1877: c. 171: First Report of the Select Committee of the House of Lords on Intemperance: Evidence of William Sproston Caine.
30. HCPP. 1877: c. 171: Evidence of William Sproston Caine.
31. HCPP. 1877: c. 171: First Report of the Select Committee of the House of Lords on Intemperance: Evidence of Alfred Eccles.
32. HCPP. 1877: c. 171: Evidence of Alfred Eccles.
33. HCPP. 1877: c. 171.
34. HCPP. 1877: c. 171: First Report of the Select Committee of the House of Lords on Intemperance: Evidence of Professor Leone Levi.

CHAPTER 4

The Secret Army of Drinkers

Of every-one hundred women who are drunk, it is probable that a larger number would commit disorderly acts, being of a more excitable temperament, and also because women when they take to evil courses are often more shameless than men?[1]

There was another group of drinkers in Victorian Britain for whom temperance and teetotalism held little weight. If working-class men can be defined as the 'great army' of drinkers then women can be regarded as the secret army, although as the quote above demonstrates, some were more secret about their drinking habits than others. The 1877 Select Committee of the House of Lords on Intemperance (1877 enquiry) investigated two main aspects of women's drinking: one was middle-class drinking linked to licensed grocers and the other was working-class drinking linked to vice and crime. The division in attitudes between public and private drinking was significant. There were many facts and figures presented regarding criminal drunkenness among poor women because they often drank publicly on the city streets and in pubs. Yet the private-drinking habits of higher-class women buying alcohol from grocers remained more elusive and often the evidence presented amounted to little more than conjecture. The standpoint of the investigation was that all women were, by their very nature, more susceptible to the effects of alcohol than men and were therefore worse drunks than men.

In the 1877 enquiry, the Chief Constable of Sheffield, John Jackson, stated that drunken arrests among women had increased from 15.7%

© The Author(s) 2018   41
T. Hands, *Drinking in Victorian and Edwardian Britain*,
https://doi.org/10.1007/978-3-319-92964-4_4

in 1847 to 24.3% in 1876.[2] When asked to account for this increase he stated that there were a higher proportion of women working in factories in Sheffield and he believed these women were adopting men's drinking habits.[3] This idea of women 'mirroring' male behaviour was a common argument put forward by many witnesses and while it did not appear to excuse women's drinking behaviour, it did locate it within the boundaries of male control. The idea that women simply mimicked men was perhaps easier to comprehend than the alternative of women actively consuming alcohol for their own purposes. Jackson argued that lower-class women more generally were more prone to drunkenness and he cited hawkers, peddlers, petty traders and factory workers as the worst drunken offenders.[4] Some committee members and witnesses seemed to share the opinion that drunken women were more of a public nuisance than drunken men and were therefore more likely to be arrested. The minister for Liverpool Prison, Reverend James Nugent, stated that in 1876 there were 4212 male prisoners and 5098 female prisoners within the gaol.[5] Moreover he stated that the majority of women were imprisoned for drink related crime and some were repeat offenders having been convicted fifty, sixty or seventy times.[6] He believed that the prison was overcrowded with women of Irish descent who lived and worked in and around the Liverpool docks making their living through prostitution.[7] Nugent described these women as ruthless in their pursuit of sailors who would provide them with shelter, clothing and drink.[8] The increase in drunken arrests among women in cities and large manufacturing towns was attributed mainly to prostitution and petty crime and often the Irish were singled out as the worst offenders.

John Bremner, a Manchester magistrate, presented statistics relating to the numbers of arrests for drunkenness among the Irish population. He stated that in 1876, the total number of drunken arrests among the Irish was 2466 and that 789 of these were women.[9] Bremner did not provide any comparative figures for previous years but did state that in 1876 the total number of drunken arrests for all women was 2743.[10] This meant that the overwhelming majority of drunken arrests were for non-Irish women. Yet this fact evaded scrutiny and instead the figures for drunken arrests among Irish women were set within the context of Bremner's views on the changing drinking habits of the Manchester working classes. He believed that a recent influx of Irish immigrants from Liverpool to Manchester to work in the cotton mills had encouraged the popularity and spread of dram shops and dancing saloons. Bremner argued that the pubs in Manchester had 'degenerated' from being houses of refreshment which served food and drink to 'simple dram shops' which encouraged female drunkenness.[11]

Many witnesses expressed the belief that women were worse drunks than men because they were more of a nuisance and more shameful. Yet it was not only witnesses who held this belief. One member of the 1877 committee, the Bishop of Carlisle commented 'I suppose the effect of liquor upon a woman is greater than upon a man; that they are more likely to be disorderly than a man would be on the same amount of liquor.'[12] This idea that women simply could not 'hold their drink' in the same way as men were put to witnesses such as general practitioners, police, prison officials and asylum doctors. Mr William Smith, Governor of Ripon Prison in Yorkshire, stated that in his experience women were prone to more frequent habits of intoxication than men.[13] He cited the example of a female prisoner who had been repeatedly convicted for drunkenness and had spent several years in and out of prison. The woman was released from prison and given a home and employment on the condition that she sign the pledge and give up drinking. The woman worked for a few weeks then she got drunk and left her job, claiming that she could not live on charity.[14] In the 1872 Select Committee on Habitual Drunkards (1872 enquiry), Dr Alexander Peddie, an Edinburgh physician noted for his professional interest in treating inebriety, recounted his experience of treating women with dipsomania

> I have had the most solemn assertions that not a drop of liquor has crossed their lips for many hours, when they could not have walked across the floor; that not a drop of liquor was within their power; when I would find bottles of liquor wrapped up in stockings and other articles of clothing … and on a late occasion, in the case of a lady, after all means had failed in discovering where the drink came from, on making a strict personal examination, found a bottle of brandy concealed in the armpit, hung around the neck with an elastic cord so that she might help herself as she pleased. Next morning seeing that the drunkenness still continued, and that something more was to be got at, there was actually found a bottle of brandy tied in some way, round the loins, and placed between her thighs.[15]

Perhaps it was Peddie's intention to provide a shocking tale of drinking that transgressed the boundaries of 'decent' and 'respectable' femininity but the idea of alcohol as a temptation that some women simply could not resist was one of the reasons why the 1877 enquiry constantly returned to the question of women and licensed grocers. The 1860 Wine and Refreshment Houses Act had led to the expansion of the off-license trade and consequently the numbers of licensed grocers selling wine, beer and spirits had increased. The 1860 Act marked Gladstone's attempts as Chancellor of the Exchequer, to overhaul the system of duties on alcohol. This involved lowering the duties on imported wine and allowing alcohol to be sold for consumption off the premises in a wider range of shops and restaurants. These measures were hoped to encourage the British population to consume wine instead of beer and spirits, which in turn was intended to promote more 'civilised' and moderate drinking habits.[16] Allowing the sale of small quantities of wine and spirits in shops and restaurants meant that alcohol could be bought from places other than pubs. Consequently, women who did not or could not visit pubs were able to buy alcohol from an increased number of retail outlets.

Many witnesses were asked about an increase in drunkenness among women that could be directly attributed to the expansion of licensed grocers. The general consensus among witnesses seemed to be that it was mainly middle-class women who purchased alcohol from grocers and that women of the lower classes were more likely to buy alcohol from pubs. Obtaining alcohol from licensed grocers was regarded as perfectly acceptable if women were buying wine and spirits for household use in dining, cooking and entertaining. However, there were concerns that some women were purchasing alcohol for their own personal use and in the 1877 enquiry, the Rector of Wrexham, Reverend David Howell stated that he knew of several instances where respectable women were led to drinking through licensed grocers. He felt that licensed grocers made it easier for women to buy liquor because they could purchase it along with their groceries, thus escaping shame and detection by their husbands.[17] Captain James Nicholls, the Chief Constable of Newcastle believed that women 'of a higher station' were inclined to purchase alcohol from grocers because they would be too ashamed to go to public houses and that grocer's licenses were directly responsible for an increase in drinking among middle and upper class women. However, when asked if he had any evidence to support his views, he stated that it was just a general opinion.[18] Witnesses often resorted to vague conjecture when asked about the links between women's drinking and licensed grocers. However, some of the evidence given during The 1878 Grocers Licenses (Scotland) Commission provided more persuasive accounts of women's drinking. The evidence from this enquiry was widely reported in the Scottish and national newspapers, providing sensationalist accounts of women's drinking. One witness, Duncan McLaren an Edinburgh MP, read an extract from the medical journal *The Lancet* that reported on a meeting of the Brewster Sessions in West Riding. Brewster sessions were the annual meetings of licensing justices to deal with the granting, renewal, and transfer of licenses to sell intoxicating liquor. The report stated that there was evidence to suggest that women who visited licensed grocers to purchase groceries were tempted to procure a bottle of wine or spirits for their own private consumption.[19] During 1877 *The Lancet* ran a series of articles relating to licensed grocers because a group of physicians, surgeons and general practitioners had signed a petition calling for parliament to look at the issue of secret drinking. In a statement published in *The Lancet* the group of 920 doctors claimed that

> We believe women, servants and children of respectable households, who could not, or would not, procure intoxicating drinks at public houses are encouraged to purchase and use these liquors by the opportunity offered when visiting grocers shops for other purposes. Female domestic servants are often enabled to obtain bottles of spirits, wine and beer at a small cost on credit, or as 'commission' on the household bills. This trade is wholly removed from police supervision and is a direct incentive to 'secret drinking' – a practice more injurious to the health and morals and social prosperity of the community than ordinary trade in intoxicating liquors.[20]

The 'evil of secret drinking' that the doctors outlined in their petition went beyond a purely medical matter because it was embroiled with ideas about respectable femininity. One witness from the Grocers Licenses (Scotland) Commission, Reverend William Turner of the Edinburgh City Mission, read a statement from one of his informers who worked for the Mission. The informer was acquainted with the daughter of a 'respectable' married woman who claimed that her mother was 'given to drink' and had purchased alcohol 'hundreds of times' from Edinburgh grocers that concealed the purchases by falsifying the customer accounts.[21] The statement continued that father of the family, described as 'a hardworking and worthy man' had checked the grocer's account books to discover that the records had been falsified to conceal his wife's purchases of whisky. The conclusion was that the grocer and the 'foolish' wife had colluded in this deceit.[22] The main dilemma facing the parliamentary enquiries and the doctors who signed the petition was deciding if licensed grocers actively encouraged, either by their very existence or in collusion with women, the practice of secret domestic drinking. This type of drinking not only challenged feminine ideals but more importantly, it defied patriarchal authority—in other words 'worthy' and 'hard working' men were being duped into paying for liquor by unscrupulous grocers and 'foolish' wives.

Yet not all the witnesses agreed that licensed grocers actively encouraged women to drink and some still felt that men largely kept women's drinking in check. One newspaper that reported on the Grocers Licenses (Scotland) Commission cited the testimony of Provost King of Rutherglen, a textile manufacturer who employed 250 women in his factory. King stated that he had no knowledge of wives drinking 'without the consent' of their husbands and therefore in this regard licensed grocers did not present any kind of temptation.[23] However it seemed that not all women sought permission from their husbands to drink. The real issue with licensed grocers was that they enabled women to drink 'in secret' beyond the male gaze. In contrast, working-class women drank publicly under the glare of moral scrutiny.

This builds a picture of female drinking that ranged across social classes and occurred in both public and private settings. Although many witnesses believed alcohol presented a temptation to women, it could be argued that it also presented a means of resisting patriarchal authority. If the great army of male drinkers stood strong against temperance and sobriety, then perhaps the women's secret army made their own stand against patriarchy and feminine ideals through the consumption of alcohol. This fits with de Certeau's ideas of a consumer grid of resistance

> Many everyday practices (talking, reading, moving about, shopping, cooking etc.) are tactical in character. And so are, more generally, many 'ways of operating': victories of the 'weak' over the 'strong' (whether the strength be that of powerful people or the violence of things or of an imposed order, etc.).[24]

Public drunkenness and secret drinking were constructed as deviant and immoral precisely because they were defiant acts that involved the agency of women as alcohol consumers. This agency held power and therefore it was difficult to grasp the concept that women could actively choose to buy and consume alcohol for their own purposes of intoxication. It was easier to locate women's drinking within the framework of patriarchy and argue that women were simply mimicking male behaviour, or shift the blame on to licensed grocers for supplying women with alcohol. The idea that women were worse drunks than men cast them as the weaker sex in terms of alcohol consumption and intoxication more broadly. Put simply, it was believed that men could handle their drink and women could not and to some extent this dictated the social rules of public and private drinking. Therefore the women who chose to drink alcohol, in spite of the social rules, were in some ways resisting the status quo.

NOTES

1. House of Commons Parliamentary Papers (HCPP). 1877: c. 171: First Report of the Select Committee of the House of Lords on Intemperance: Question from Lord Aberdaire to John Jackson, Chief Constable of Sheffield.
2. HCPP. 1877: c. 171: First Report from the Select Committee of the House of Lords on Intemperance: Evidence of John Jackson, Chief Constable of Sheffield.
3. HCPP. 1877: c. 171: First Report from the Select Committee of the House of Lords on Intemperance: Evidence of John Jackson, Chief Constable of Sheffield.
4. HCPP. 1877: c. 171: First Report from the Select Committee of the House of Lords on Intemperance: Evidence of John Jackson, Chief Constable of Sheffield.
5. HCPP. 1877: c. 418: Third Report of the Select Committee of the House of Lords on Intemperance: Evidence of Reverend James Nugent.
6. HCPP. 1877: c. 418: Third Report of the Select Committee of the House of Lords on Intemperance: Evidence of Reverend James Nugent.
7. HCPP. 1877: c. 418: Third Report of the Select Committee of the House of Lords on Intemperance: Evidence of Reverend James Nugent.
8. HCPP. 1877: c. 418: Evidence of Reverend James Nugent.
9. HCPP. 1877: c. 271: Second Report of the Select Committee of the House of Lords on Intemperance: Evidence of John Alexander Bremner.
10. HCPP. 1877: c. 271: Evidence of John Alexander Bremner.
11. HCPP. 1877: c. 271: Evidence of John Alexander Bremner.
12. HCPP. 1877: c. 418: Third Report of the Select Committee of the House of Lords on Intemperance: Evidence of Reverend James Nugent: Question from the Bishop of Carlisle to Reverend Nugent.
13. HCPP. 1877: c. 271: Second Report of the Select Committee of the House of Lords on Intemperance: Evidence of Mr William Smith.

14. HCPP. 1877: c. 271: Evidence of Mr William Smith.
15. HCPP. 1872: c. 242: Select Committee on Habitual Drunkards: Evidence of Dr Alexander Peddie.
16. Briggs A. 1985. *Wine for Sale: Victoria Wine and the Liquor Trade 1860–1914*: Chicago: University of Chicago Press: pp. 9–18.
17. HCPP. 1877: c. 418: Third Report of the Select Committee of the House of Lords on Intemperance: Evidence of Reverend David Howell.
18. HCPP. 1877: c. 271: Second Report of the Select Committee of the House of Lords on Intemperance: Evidence of Captain James Nicholls.
19. HCPP. 1878: c. 1941: Grocers Licenses (Scotland) Commission: Evidence of Duncan McLaren MP.
20. 'The Grocers License', *The Lancet*: Volume 110:2810: 7 July 1877: pp. 27–18.
21. HCPP. 1878: c. 1941: Grocers Licenses (Scotland) Commission: Evidence of Reverend William Turner.
22. HCPP. 1878: c. 1941: Grocers Licenses (Scotland) Commission: Evidence of Reverend William Turner.
23. 'Royal Commission on Licensed Grocers': *The Glasgow Herald*: 25 October 1877.
24. de Certeau M. 1984. *The Practice of Everyday Life*: Berkeley: University of California Press: p. xix.

CHAPTER 5

Testing the 'Character of Drink'

There were many references made throughout the parliamentary enquiries to the type of alcohol sold and consumed within pubs and other drinking places because different types and qualities of alcohol were believed to influence drinking behaviour. The quality of beer, wine and spirits varied enormously and some brewers and publicans used adulterants to enhance the quality, taste or strength of the liquor sold.[1] Joseph Chamberlain read a statement from a Birmingham chemical analyst who had been commissioned to examine the beer sold in certain 'low class' public houses

> The samples are all very dark in colour, of a harsh disagreeable taste, and unusually bitter. The character of the bitter, which clung persistently to the palate, is altogether unlike the pleasant, transient, aromatic flavour of the hop, of which I believe all, or nearly all, the samples to be entirely innocent. I drank some of each sample and found them all heady in their effects and seemed to dispose of diarrhoea. I have however been unable, by either chemical or other tests to prove the presence of coccolus indicus.[2]

Chamberlain stated that in his opinion, many of the problems of drunkenness could be eradicated by changing 'the character of the drink which the population consumes.'[3] Moreover, he believed that the poorer working classes were so used to consuming poor quality beer that they offered 'Bass's best beer' they would refuse it because the strength of the beer sold in lower-class pubs matched that of spirits such as brandy.[4]

© The Author(s) 2018
T. Hands, *Drinking in Victorian and Edwardian Britain*,
https://doi.org/10.1007/978-3-319-92964-4_5

Chamberlain and other witnesses believed that the problems of intemperance extended beyond the types of drinkers or amounts of alcohol consumed to encompass the type and quality of alcohol that was sold to the population.

In the late nineteenth century alcohol was produced on an industrial scale in Britain and those involved in the drink trade benefitted from advances in science and technology that increased productivity and maximised profits. Although this meant wider choice and cheaper prices for alcohol consumers, there were concerns at a political level regarding the quality of alcohol that was sold to the public. Chamberlain stated that the Birmingham analyst strongly suspected the presence of the drug cocculus indicus (an intoxicant added to boost the strength of weak beer) and that in his opinion, certain lower-class pubs were selling beer that was 'unduly intoxicating and unwholesome and quite different from genuine ales.[5] As Burns notes there was a 'general climate of adulteration' in the late nineteenth century and it was common practice for manufacturers and publicans to add a range of additives to food and drink to either improve the taste or to extract more profit.[6] Some of these additives were legal and fairly benign in nature but others were potentially toxic and posed a risk to health. The main reasons that manufacturers and publicans had for adulterating alcohol were to improve the taste, appearance and strength of watered down or poor quality beer and spirits or to enhance the taste of 'silent' or 'foreign' spirits that were sold to the public as 'genuine' spirits. Although the 1872 Licensing Act made it an offence to keep or sell adulterated liquor, the practice was still widespread because detection and prosecution were difficult and some publicans were intent on boosting profits with the help of water and chemical additives.[7]

The adulteration of beer by publicans was one concern that featured throughout the parliamentary enquiries. However there was often more attention given to adulterated spirits because of the higher levels of alcohol and intoxication. The 1890 Select Committee on British and Foreign spirits looked at the issue of adulteration and heard evidence from witnesses such as Inland Revenue officials and chemical analysts. The enquiry was concerned with investigating three key issues regarding the production, sale and consumption of spirits in Britain: First was the bonding of spirits for maturity and whether this practice should be made compulsory to ensure the sale of better quality spirits. Second was the blending of spirits produced by patent and pot still distillation derived from different countries of origin and whether this practice was in the best interests of alcohol consumers. There were questions about the possible health implications of blending spirits and also over the labelling of blended spirits that were composed of different substances. The third issue under investigation was the consumption of intoxicants such as ether, methylated spirits and 'new' spirits that had not been matured and what impact these substances had on public health. The enquiry was conducted with a scientific rigour and chemical analysts were summoned to provide evidence on the distillation process and chemical composition of spirits. The subject of fusel oil featured prominently throughout the enquiry. Fusel oil was a generic name given to a range of chemical constituents sometimes referred to as 'impurities' which were produced by spirit distillation and included amyl-alcohol and other oily compounds. Fusel oil was believed to be present in different amounts and compositions in many alcoholic drinks. It was the amount of fusel oil present that mattered because it was believed to affect the quality and taste of spirits and also the health and behaviour of consumers.

The enquiry heard evidence from two analytical chemists employed by the Inland Revenue and the Board of Customs. These men tested various samples of spirits obtained from distilleries and pubs in order to assess the extent to which methods of distillation and the process of blending and bonding spirits affected the quality, purity, strength and taste of spirits sold to the public. Dr Bell, Principal Chemist of the Inland Revenue Laboratory obtained 51 samples of spirits from working-class pubs situated in the 'lowest parts' of towns in England, Ireland and Scotland. Bell subjected the samples to a chemical analysis and a taste test, which he concluded was 'satisfactory'.[8] He reported that the spirits sold in public houses were highly rectified (distilled) and of good quality and strength which was indicative of patent still distillation methods. This produced cheap, commercially viable spirits such as gin and whisky but also produced a 'silent spirit' or 'German spirit'[9] that could be mixed with other alcoholic drinks such as brandy, whisky and sherry to produce 'fake' spirits. Bell argued that from his perspective as a chemist cheap patent still spirits and 'fake' spirits were of a sufficient quality, strength and purity to pose no hazard to public health. However the Committee were not satisfied with his conclusions and pressed him to state for the record if he believed that 'fake' French brandy, Scotch whisky or West Indian rum were better than the genuine articles.[10] Bell stated that the preference for 'fake' or 'real' spirits was purely a matter of consumer taste and that in his opinion the public preferred less highly flavoured spirits produced by patent still production and by blending cheap 'silent' spirit with more expensive 'real' spirits.[11] Bell gave the impression that he did not think the public were being duped either in terms of taste or quality by cheap, mass produced blended spirits. However, the persistent line of questioning from the Committee suggested that they thought otherwise.

At one point the committee presented Bell with a glass of Scotch and a glass of Irish whisky purchased from the House of Commons bar. Bell was asked to test the whiskies in order to establish their point of origin—i.e. patent or pot still distillation and to test the quality and purity of the drinks. In 1890 James Buchanan & Co. had the contract to sell blended Scotch whisky in the Houses of Parliament so presumably the glass of Scotch was Buchanan's blended whisky and the glass of Irish whisky was most likely a single malt whisky produced by traditional pot still methods. This whisky test was seemingly conducted in order to aid the committee's deliberations over the correct labelling of spirits and to establish if labels should state the country of origin. However, the line of questioning leading up to the whisky test constantly pressed Bell for his opinions on which types of alcohol were 'better'—British or foreign, patent or pot still, blended or single malt whiskies, bonded or 'new' spirits.[12] There was a sense that the committee members were approaching the subject not only from a political standpoint but also as alcohol consumers. They were either reluctant to accept Bell's view that there was little difference in the quality of single malt or blended whisky or perhaps they just wanted to know exactly what they were drinking.

The second analytical chemist that gave evidence to the 1890 enquiry was Mr Cobden Samuel, the principal analyst of the Customs Laboratory. Cobden Samuel conducted experiments on himself using samples of spirits containing different levels of fusel oils in order to investigate the physical effects of drinking spirits produced by different distillation and blending methods. Over a period of days he regularly consumed quantities of 'genuine' 15-year-old brandy to which he added commercial fusel oil. He reported no ill effects and stated that his appetite and urine were normal. He then consumed quantities of 'pure' spirits with little or no fusel oil or 'impurities' present and reported that after a few days he began to feel unwell and suffered frequent headaches, tightness in the chest and acute attacks of indigestion.[13] He, therefore, concluded that 'plain' or 'silent' spirits were in fact injurious to health in their pure form and that the presence of 'impurities' or fusels oil in spirits was beneficial not only in terms of health but also in terms of the quality and taste of spirits. Cobden Samuel essentially refuted Bell's evidence by arguing that 'genuine' spirits containing fusel oil and impurities produced by traditional methods, were better for health than 'fake' or 'silent' spirits produced by commercial patent still methods. Cobden Samuel attributed the headaches he experienced after drinking silent spirits to the 'maddening' effects of new spirits which were believed to produce erratic, volatile and sometimes violent behaviour.[14]

The links between alcohol consumption and behaviour was a common theme throughout the parliamentary enquiries. Many witnesses believed that the cheap alcohol sold and consumed in lower working class areas was either adulterated beer or mass produced poor quality spirits and the effects of consumption were drunken and sometimes violent or criminal behaviour. The committees often returned to questions about certain types of alcohol inducing more or less drunkenness and whether there were any medical benefits to be gained from moderate drinking. At the 1877 enquiry, Thomas Lauder Brunton, a doctor and lecturer in Materia Medica at St Bartholomew's Hospital in London was asked if he believed that a glass of wine or spirits taken in moderation might be useful in the case of impaired digestion. He agreed that it was very useful and that: 'a man working hard all day has an exhausted stomach that is slow to digest food and a glass of wine speeds digestion'.[15] Brunton also stated that alcohol was a useful medicine in treating fevers and as an aid to insomnia. When asked about the types of alcohol used by doctors Brunton stated that he prescribed only 'good wine' or 'pure wine' because these left no bad effects afterwards.[16] Another doctor that gave evidence was Sir William Gull who was consulting physician at Guy's Hospital in London. Gull was asked if he would recommend that men working outdoors in hard physical labour should consume small amounts of 'nutritious light beer.' and replied

> I think some stomachs have more power to consume common food, while others want food more highly prepared. I do not think at present, from our knowledge, we should be prepared to say that everybody could go without beer. It is a food of a light kind.[17]

Although Gull believed that working-class labourers benefitted from consuming moderate amounts of beer, he disagreed with one committee member's suggestion that intellectual work also required alcohol and stated that in his opinion moderate consumption harmed the nervous systems and brains of the higher classes.[18] Like the 1890 enquiry, the line of questioning often veered from impartiality and exposed the concerns of committee members as alcohol consumers. It is reasonable to assume that most committee members drank alcohol for various reasons—either to relax and socialise, for health reasons or to combat fatigue and 'stimulate' intellectual output. It is also likely that aside from the fervent pro-temperance supporters, many witnesses were regular drinkers and their opinions on their own drinking habits and those of others were coloured by their experiences as alcohol consumers. In this sense, professionalism and impartiality often gave way to the personal opinions and anecdotal evidence of alcohol consumers.

NOTES

1. Burns E. 1995. *Bad Whisky.* Glasgow: Balvag Books: p. 10.
2. House of Commons Parliamentary Papers (HCPP). c. 171: First Report of the Select Committee of the House of Lords on Intemperance: Evidence of Joseph Chamberlain.
3. Ibid.
4. Ibid.
5. HCPP. c. 171: First Report of the Select Committee of the House of Lords on Intemperance: Evidence of Joseph Chamberlain.
6. Burns: p. 13.
7. Ibid.: p. 32.
8. HCPP. c. 316: First Report of the Select Committee on British and Foreign Spirits: Evidence of Dr Bell.
9. Patent still spirit was often imported from abroad and the name 'German spirit' was applied to any imported spirit although most were imported from Russia.
10. HCPP. c. 316: First Report of the Select Committee on British and Foreign Spirits: Evidence of Dr Bell.
11. Ibid.
12. HCPP. c. 316: First Report of the Select Committee on British and Foreign Spirits: Evidence of Dr Bell.
13. HCPP. c. 316: First Report of the Select Committee on British and Foreign Spirits: Evidence of Mr Cobden Samuel.
14. HCPP. c. 316: First Report of the Select Committee on British and Foreign Spirits: Evidence of Mr Cobden Samuel.

15. HCPP. c. 418: Third report of the Select Committee on Intemperance: Evidence of Thomas Lauder Brunton.
16. Ibid.
17. HCPP. c. 418: Third report of the Select Committee on Intemperance: Evidence of Sir William Gull.
18. Ibid.

PART II

Drinks

This part provides three case studies of Victorian alcohol producers and retailers: Bass & Co, a major brewer based in Burton-upon-Trent; whisky producers James Buchanan and John Walker whose companies expanded the market for Scotch whisky in England and W & A Gilbey, one of the leading wine and spirit merchants in the late nineteenth century. Each of these companies operated in an increasingly competitive market for alcoholic drinks. It was therefore necessary to adapt business models and commercial practices to secure profits from the sale of wines, beers and spirits. Although each case study tells a different story, they share some commonalities. Each company realised that selling alcohol in late Victorian Britain required a degree of cunning, ingenuity and a leap of imagination in order to circumvent temperance ideology and reach an expanding consumer market. People did not need to be given reasons to drink—despite decades of the Temperance Movement, many continued to do so. However there was profit to be made in marketing alcohol as a socially acceptable (and sometimes desirable) drink that not only had health-giving properties but also embodied British cultural ideals.

CHAPTER 6

Selling 'the Drink of the Empire': Bass & Co. Ltd

It is easy to see why pale, bitter ale made great headway in the 1840-1900 period, the golden age of British beer drinking. It was novel, bright, fresh and pale; it looked good in the new glassware; it was the high fashion of beer of the railway age. Perfected in Burton, it was, by the 1870s, produced everywhere.[1]

Tastes in beer changed during the nineteenth century and this was driven in part by the expansion of the brewing industry and also by changing social attitudes and leisure pursuits.[2] Although regional breweries continued to produce a variety of beers that catered to local markets, one of the key national changes was a general shift in tastes from strong dark beers and porter to light sparkling beers and ales. This is largely attributed to the expansion of the brewing industry in Burton upon Trent in the 1840s which was driven by the development of India Pale Ale (IPA).[3] Burton brewers, Allsopp and Bass began developing a heavily hopped, pale bitter beer for the Indian export market in the 1820s. IPA was developed to survive long sea voyages and hot climates and was therefore a successful export commodity to India and the colonies. Foster attributes the commercial success of IPA not only to its robust qualities, which made it a safe and pleasant alternative to local drinking water but also because for colonists, it evoked ideas about Britishness.[4]

The development of IPA and can be traced to the October ales which were produced in the seventeenth and eighteenth centuries. Beer production was closely aligned with the agricultural seasons and the beers

© The Author(s) 2018
T. Hands, *Drinking in Victorian and Edwardian Britain*,
https://doi.org/10.1007/978-3-319-92964-4_6

brewed at the beginning of the season used the freshest hops and malt right after the autumn harvest. The practice of using exclusively pale malt was expensive and was therefore usually found among country estate brewers who catered to the wealthiest country gentry.[5] By the mid-eighteenth century, commercial brewers in London were also producing pale beers alongside darker beers and porter. However, pale beer was more expensive and was therefore viewed as a status drink which was popular among the upper classes, many of who became colonists in India. The market for pale ales was closely linked to the expansion of the British Empire and also to the spread of imperial ideology. This was one of the key reasons for the commercial success of Bass & Co. which produced and exported the largest volume of IPA in the late nineteenth century.

Following the railway expansion in the 1840s, the Burton brewers began to develop variants of IPA for the domestic market. Up until that point IPA had not been sold in Britain and although it is likely that the Burton brewers seized upon a commercial opportunity to cultivate domestic tastes for pale ale, a more exciting story circulating at the time claimed that a ship carrying a cargo of IPA destined for India was shipwrecked in the Irish Sea and the cargo was salvaged and sold off in Liverpool where local drinkers sampled it and liked the taste.[6] As Jonathan Reinarz notes, 'shipwreck theory' provides an attractive explanation for the commercial success of IPA because it supports the prevalent historical view that nineteenth-century brewers spent very little time or resources on marketing and advertising.[7] The Bass records support the idea that there was more to the commercial success of pale ale than simply 'success by chance.' In fact, the larger Burton brewers such as Bass & Co., spent considerable amounts of money on advertising pale ale and expanding the domestic market for its products.

Bass brewery was a family business established in Burton upon Trent in the 1770s. The company initially supplied local pubs and inns in the surrounding areas. Then in the late eighteenth century, it merged with another local brewer, Samuel Ratcliff and together they built a strong export trade to the Baltic region. When the Baltic trade began to fail after 1800, the company again merged with another local brewer John Gretton and trading as 'Bass, Ratcliff and Gretton' turned its attention to cultivating trade links to India and the colonies by developing and exporting IPA.[8] The company also extended its reach into the domestic market. Between 1850 and 1880 25% of beer and ale sales went to the London market; 18% were exported; 22% were distributed locally and 35% were sold by other agencies.[9] By the 1880s, Bass was producing approximately 850,000 barrels per year with the production of pale ale accounting for 56% of total output.[10] The company also secured its share of the domestic market through the tied house system and by buying licensed premises in Burton and surrounding areas and in London.[11]

When Alfred Barnard visited Bass & Co. in 1889, he described the brewery as a major part of Burton's 'beer metropolis.'[12] Barnard was a journalist with a particular interest in the drink trade. He published detailed accounts of his tours around various breweries in Britain and Ireland and seemed to be particularly impressed with the production site at Bass & Co. where he found that 'a steady and undeviating perseverance of uniformity, order and regularity, is discernible in all the buildings and breweries connected with Bass & Co.'s establishment.'[13] The detail in Barnard's account conveys the sheer enormity of the Bass production site which included 12 miles of railway track connecting all the buildings in the company grounds. Barnard was clearly impressed with the production process which used modern brewing equipment and employed analytical chemists to test and enhance the quality of products. This was brewing on a truly modern and industrial scale. However, the volume of output was not enough to maintain and promote the company's share of the market. It was, therefore, important to create a distinct brand identity that would be associated with all Bass products. During his tour, Barnard visited the bottle-labelling department, which he described as

… a large and important one in this establishment. [It] is conducted by a Superintendent and several clerks. The well-known red triangle or pyramid, in the centre of the oval label, used for Bass & Co.'s bottled pale ale is one of their numerous trademarks and has been in use by them for upwards of fifty years.[14]

The red triangle or 'pyramid' and the red diamond were in fact the first British company trademarks to be registered under the Trade Marks Registration Act in 1842. Bass was aware of the need to protect the brand identity and the company kept a label book which contained various Bass labels and those used by rival companies. This book contained labels from c. 1870 to 1924 which appear to have been used as a means of keeping a record of the development of new product labelling and also of any attempts by rival companies to copy Bass product branding.

Bass also kept an Infringement Book which contained evidence of any fraudulent attempts to copy or use Bass product branding. One undated entry in the book titled 'Bass & Co.'s advertisements—case to advise' stated

> Bass, Ratcliff and Gretton Ltd are the owners of a trademark in the form of a triangle which is coloured red. Certain public houses where their beer is to be obtained have painted on the window adjoining the public house the triangle and in some cases there is the addition of 'Bass & Co.'s Ales' too ... Strangers seeing the mark on the windows are drawn into the house under the impression that they can obtain Bass & Co. ale. We have no evidence as to whether they ask for Bass & Co. ale and are supplied in draught or in bottle with ale either by no remark being made as to whether it is Bass & Co. or not, but there is no doubt that keeping up the mark attracts customers.[15]

The company invested considerable time and resources in order to protect the brand from fraudulent use. An online search of the British Newspaper Archive for 'Bass Pale Ale labels' (1850–1900) generated numerous reports of prosecutions for false labelling of products. For example, in 1859 *The Belfast Morning News* reported the case of a local wine and spirit merchant charged with purchasing quantities of pale ale and falsely labelling the bottles with an imitation Bass logo.[16] Another similar case reported in *The Manchester Courier* in 1886 was of a local ale and porter merchant charged with putting false Bass labels on his products.[17] In each of these cases Bass & Co. successfully pursued legal action against the individuals that had attempted to use the Bass logo. The company also placed adverts in newspapers warning customers to be wary of false labelling on products claiming to be Bass Pale Ale and recommended that customers deface the labels on empty bottles to prevent them from being refilled with 'inferior' ale.[18] By making such a public spectacle of protecting the brand image, the company not only dissuaded fraudulent activity but more importantly, it sent out a clear message to consumers that Bass was a reputable company selling high-quality products that were worth protecting. Although tracking down and prosecuting fraudsters may have been time-consuming and expensive, ultimately it enhanced the company image which in turn made the Bass brand even more exclusive and desirable.

Although the origins of the red triangle design are somewhat unclear, it grew to symbolise quality and authenticity. Some historical accounts state that a clerk at Bass & Co. created the red triangle design in 1855.[19] The reasoning behind the design is less clear. The Bass company scrapbook contained an amusing clip from *The Westminster Gazette* in 1894, which claimed that

> Everybody knows the red pyramid pale ale label surrounded by a Staffordshire knot. It was the design of Mr George Curzon, one of the employees in the London agency and was first used in 1855. Some years ago an ingenious writer in one of the Sheffield papers wittily invented a classical legend about this label ... the pyramid builders worshipped a great power called by some Tammuz, by others Bassareus, the son of the goddess Ops. He was termed Bassareus the fortifier ...[20]

It is perhaps more likely that the triangle design represented the three key elements in Bass & Co.—namely, Bass, Ratcliff and Gretton or that the company realized the potential to reach consumers by using a simple bold geometric design on product labelling. In any case, a distinct brand image ensured that Bass products were visible during a period of intense competition in the foreign and domestic markets for beer. As Table 6.1 shows, the company spent increasing amounts on product labelling and advertising around the turn of the century

By 1904, the advertising budget had grown in line with the company profit from sales, which increased from £3,102,479 in 1895 to £3,642,377 in 1904.[21] At this time the company had an extensive system of agencies in various cities around the UK and the world. Between 1902 and 1903, sales increases were reported in Bristol, Nottingham, Glasgow, Belfast, Plymouth, Exeter, New York and Paris.[22] Indeed, by the late nineteenth century, Bass Pale Ale had even penetrated Parisian bohemian culture.

Table 6.1 Bass & Co. balance sheets 1896–1904.[23]

Show cards, labels & stationery	Expenses
1896	£13,939 7s 8d
1897	£17,762 18s 2d
1898	£23,086 13s 2d
1899	£26,284 10s 2d
1900	£22,373 1s 11d
1901	£24,232 9s 9d
1902	£20,945 3s 4d
1903	£27,779 8s 4d
1904	£39,321 4s 6d

Edouard Manet's impressionist painting from 1882 features bottles of Bass No. 1 Pale Ale on prominent display on the bar of the Folies-Bergere, which was one of Paris' top music hall venues frequented by Manet and other artists.

Although Bass had cultivated a market for its products in Paris, the sales book for 1902–1903 also noted a marked decrease in sales in London and Newcastle. Between 1903 and 1905 profits from sales also dropped from £3,866,320 to £3,481,131.[24] This decline in domestic sales followed the passing of The 1902 Licensing Act which imposed restrictions on the granting of new pub licenses. Since Bass had an extensive network of tied houses and had paid loans to many pubs, hotels and railway hotels across England, the decline in domestic sales and profits could be partly attributed to the change in legislation. It would, therefore, have been important to generate new sales and a key way to reach consumers was through advertising.

Bass had already established a strong brand image through product labelling and by the turn of the century, the company had built a reputation for selling high-quality beers and ales. Dwindling sales meant that in order to reach more consumers it was necessary to 'invent' new reasons for drinking Bass products and to sell these ideas to consumers— in essence, give people more reasons to drink Bass products. In order to be commercially successful, these reasons had to reflect cultural values and ideally reinforce them. One example was an advert from 1911 which depicted Bass's 'world-famed' pale ale as 'The Drink of the Empire' with its path to success from 1778 to 1911 closely mirroring the expansion and dominance of the British empire. Whether intentional or not, there certainly seemed to be some truth in this advert. In the eighteenth century, pale (or October) ale was the drink favoured by the landed gentry, colonists and military elites. It was a socially desirable drink before it was exported to the colonies and became IPA. The conflation of ideas about social class and British imperialism was already part of the appeal of the drink. All Bass had to do was market those ideas.

Bass advertising also drew upon on other aspects of British culture such as the practice of 'having a nip' of alcohol to keep out the cold winter weather or to 'ward off chills'. Bass ale was promoted as 'the best winter drink' because it contained 'nourishing' qualities which were not found in spirits. These adverts had a twofold purpose: to promote the idea that beer had health-giving properties and to persuade consumers that more expensive beers, like Bass, were especially therapeutic. It was important that consumers viewed beer as a viable alternative to the 'pick-me-up' offered by tonic wines and cheap spirits. Bass ales, although more expensive, had a reputation as medicinal alcoholic drinks that were prescribed by the medical profession.

In 1852, several articles on the chemical composition of Burton ales appeared in *The Lancet*. These followed reports from a chemist in France, that British bitter ales contained quantities of strychnine. As the reports were circulated in the British press, Allsopp and Bass grew concerned and asked *The Lancet* to conduct chemical analyses of their beers and to publish the results in the journal. It is clear from the extract of the report shown below that *The Lancet* undertook the task of analysing the beers not only because the medical profession prescribed (and perhaps drank) Burton ales but also because the French dared to attack the British national drink.

In all those countries in which the vine tree is extensively cultivated, wine is the ordinary beverage of the population; while in England the climate being unsuited to the growth of the vine, beer is the national beverage and enters into daily consumption of all classes of persons, from the richest to the poorest. It is therefore not extraordinary that any statement calculated to throw a suspicion on the genuine character of beer, should be viewed with alarm by the public and with the utmost concern by those engaged in the manufacture, whose pecuniary interests are of course largely involved.[25]

The reports provided very favourable analyses of Bass pale ale and IPA and refuted any claims that 'British beers' contained strychnine. Indeed, the reports also did a very good job of advertising the therapeutic qualities of Bass products

From the pure and wholesome nature of the ingredients employed, the moderate proportion of alcohol present and the very considerable quantity of aromatic anodyne bitter derived from the hops contained in these beers, they tend to preserve the tone and rigour of the stomach and conduce the restoration of the health of that organ when in a state of weakness or debility ... it is very satisfactory to find that a beverage of such general consumption is entirely free from any kind of impurity.[26]

Although these reports appeared before the height of medical temperance later in the century when the medical profession shied away from such unreserved endorsements of the medicinal qualities of alcohol, they do highlight one of the key ways in which Bass ales came to be regarded as 'wholesome' national drinks. Half a century later, Bass marketed 'barley wine' (which was in fact a high gravity heavily malted beer) as a 'wholesome' medicinal winter drink. One advert for barley wine used another report from *The Lancet* which once again analysed the chemical composition of a Bass product and found that it possessed 'a decidedly nourishing value' compared to other strong beers and stouts.[27] This medical endorsement would undoubtedly have helped Bass to market a higher alcohol beer as a viable alternative to other popular 'medicinal' drinks like invalid stouts, tonic wines and of course spirits like brandy and whisky.

By the turn of the century, Bass was one of many companies competing in the growing domestic market for alcoholic 'health' drinks and many of the adverts from the 1890–1910 period drew upon concepts of beer as a nutritious medicinal drink that could be used in a variety of situations for an array of health complaints. One advertising campaign used the miseries of the daily grind to convince consumers that Bass ale could help cure their ills. These adverts posed questions such as: 'Can't eat? Can't sleep?' and 'Too tired to sleep?' or 'Tired or run down?'—and in every case the answer to the problem was to be found in a 'nutritious' glass of Bass ale. Another way to reach consumers was to market products for home consumption. This was undoubtedly a wise move during a period when restrictive licensing, limited pub opening hours and moral judgments made the trip to the local pub difficult or impossible for certain groups, most notably women.

By the early twentieth century, dwindling sales meant that it was important to reach and indeed create new groups of consumers whose custom and loyalty demanded more than a strong brand image. Creating and securing this market meant giving people 'good reasons' to drink Bass products—for health; to combat the daily grind of work or to cope with the worst of the British weather. Perhaps, people already drank beer for these reasons and all that Bass had to do was market these uses and sell the idea that Bass products were a cure-all for illness or an antidote to the stresses and strains of modern life. Intoxication was not marketed as a 'good reason' to drink Bass beer; in fact, the advertising was designed to draw consumers away from the very notion of intoxication—why drink to get drunk when there were so many other reasons to drink beer? Jean Baudrillard considers the manufacturing of needs and desires through the practices of marketing and advertising and argues that ideas about commodities are often unrelated to their primary function.[28] In this sense, commodities communicate particular ideas about a society by creating and reinforcing cultural values. Alcohol acts as an intoxicant but the state of intoxication (drunkenness) was socially undesirable and therefore, it was necessary to market alcohol as a sign of something else: health; wellbeing; sociability; Britishness—or perhaps wealth, status and privilege. When King Edward VII visited the Bass site in 1902, the company seized upon the opportunity to publicise the event by marketing a special brew called 'King's Ale' which was also known as 'Bass No. 1 Strong Ale'. This kind of elite endorsement was something that drove the fortunes of another major alcohol producer in the late Victorian period, James Buchanan & Co. Ltd.

NOTES

1. Wilson R. G. 1988. 'The Changing Taste for Beer in Victorian Britain', in (eds.) Wilson R. G. and Gourvish T. R. *The Dynamics of the International Brewing Industry Since 1800*: London: Routledge: p. 99.
2. Ibid.: pp. 93–105.
3. Ibid.
4. Foster T. 1990. *Pale Ale*, U.S.: Brewers Publications: p. 11.
5. Houghland J. E. 2014. 'The Origins and Diaspora of the IPA', in (eds.) Patterson M. and Hoalst-Pullen N. *The Geography of Beer: Regions, Environment & Societies*: New York: Springer: pp. 119–131.
6. Ibid.
7. Reinarz J. 2007. 'Promoting the Pint: Ale and Advertising in Late Victorian and Edwardian England': *Social History of Alcohol and Drugs*: Volume 22:1: p. 26.
8. Owen C. 1992. *The Greatest Brewery in the World: A History of Bass, Ratcliff and Gretton*: Chesterfield: Derbyshire Record Society.
9. Ibid.: pp. 77–78.
10. Ibid.
11. Ibid.: p. 27.
12. Barnard A. 1889. *Noted Breweries of Great Britain and Ireland Volume 1*: London: Joseph Carlson & Sons: p. 46.
13. Ibid.: p. 49.
14. Ibid.: p. 117.
15. National Brewery Archive (NBA), Bass & Co. Infringement Book 1870–1925.
16. *The Belfast Morning News*: 3 March 1859.
17. *The Manchester Courier*: 23 May 1886.

18. *Northern Whig*: 'Bass's Pale Ale: Caution Notice': 21 March 1863.
19. Owen C. 1992. *The Greatest Brewery in the World: A History of Bass, Ratcliff and Gretton*: Chesterfield: Derbyshire Record Society; Barnard A. 1889. *Noted Breweries of Great Britain and Ireland Volume 1*: London: Joseph Carlson & Sons.
20. NBA: M/5/33: Bass Scrapbook: *The Westminster Gazette*: 31 January 1894.
21. NBA: Bass, Ratcliff & Gretton Ltd Balance Sheets: 1895–1904: Income from sales of ale, stout and sundry products.
22. NBA: B1/18: Bass & Co. Ltd Comparative Agency Sales Book: 1902–1903.
23. NBA: A/100: Bass, Ratcliff & Gretton Ltd, Balance Sheets: 1896–1904.
24. NBA: Bass, Ratcliff & Gretton Ltd Balance Sheets: 1895–1914: Income from sales of ale, stout and sundry products.
25. 'Records of the Results of the Microscopical and Chemical Analyses of the Solids and Fluids Consumed by all Classes of the Public: The Bitter Beer, Pale Ale and India Pale Ale of Messrs Allsopp & Sons and Messrs Bass & Co of Burton Upon Trent': *The Lancet*: Volume 59:1498: 15 May 1852: pp. 473–477.
26. 'Analyses of the Bitter Beer and Indian Pale Ales Brewed by Messrs Bass & Co.': *The Lancet*: Volume 1:1498: 15 May 1852: pp. 478–479.
27. An extract of the 1909 article is shown below on the product label.
28. Baudrillard J. 1988. 'Consumer Society', in (ed.) Poster M. *Selected Writings*: Cambridge: Polity Press: pp. 29–56.

CHAPTER 7

Making Scotch Respectable: Buchanan and Walker

Many were aware of whisky's shortcomings and idiosyncrasies. Grain whiskies were smooth but dull. Malts had flavour and charisma, but varied from batch to batch. The solution was blended whisky which combined grain and malt and ironed out their inconsistencies to give a consistently good drink.[1]

The trade in blended whisky expanded in the second half of the nineteenth century. This was the period of the so-called 'whisky tide' when Scotch whisky became a popular drink south of the border. Spiller believes that the popularity of Scotch whisky is linked to Walter Scott romanticism, the growth in Highland tourism and the grouse season attracting high society.[2] The idea of a good Scotch was appealing but as the quote above suggests, the quality and taste of single malt or grain whiskies varied. Several key events led to the growth and development of the trade in blended whisky in the second half of the nineteenth century. The spread of the railway system in the 1850s had opened up the English market to Scottish products more generally.[3] The trade in whisky expanded after the passing of The 1860 Spirits Act which allowed the blending of spirits in bonded warehouses without the payment of duty. The initial purpose of whisky blending was to reduce the cost of pure malt by mixing it with cheaper grain spirit made using the patent still method. In 1865, The Scotch Distillers Association was formed through an amalgamation of six major distillers looking to secure the future of their businesses by regulating the price and output of grain whisky.[4]

© The Author(s) 2018
T. Hands, *Drinking in Victorian and Edwardian Britain*,
https://doi.org/10.1007/978-3-319-92964-4_7

As Ronald Weir notes, between 1870 and 1914, distillers operated in a highly competitive free trade environment.[5] In 1870, the total output of home-produced spirits was 24.4 million proof gallons (mpg) and this rose in 1900 to a total output of 42.8 mpg.[6]

These events occurred around the same time as the Phylloxera plant disease wiped out an estimated one-third to a half of French vineyards. This impacted upon the availability of brandy in England and thus created a niche in the market for the sale of whisky. Brandy was the preferred drink of the middle-and upper-classes and therefore in order to fill the gap in the brandy market, whisky had to be marketed as a suitable replacement and had to appeal to the tastes of English consumers. Spanish sherry was another popular drink in the nineteenth century and it was common for empty sherry barrels to be used by distillers to mature whisky. Consequently, the whisky matured in sherry barrels tasted like brandy.[7] By the 1890s, there was large-scale production of blended whiskies in Scotland which led to increased competition in both the domestic and foreign markets for whisky. Successful companies like Buchanan, Dewar and Walker (known as 'the big three') made their fortunes from the production and sale of blended whiskies that were developed primarily for the English market. The success of these products rested in part on the skill of blenders to create Scotch that suited the English palate and also on the ability of companies to market scotch as a viable alternative to brandy that would appeal to the middle-and upper-classes.

The transformation of an ordinary commodity like blended whisky into Scotch, which became a status drink among the social elites, involved targeting specific groups of consumers and selling them particular ideas about the substance and James Buchanan did this very successfully. When Buchanan (who became Lord Woolavington) died in 1935, the *Daily Express* ran his obituary with the headline: 'The secret that made Lord Woolavington: He found the formula for making England like Scotch Whisky.' The article went on to report that Lord Woolavington had the reputation of being the wealthiest of the great whisky distillers of modern times. He started work as a clerk and the secret of his success was he found a formula for making Scotch whisky that was palatable to Englishmen.[8] James Buchanan (1849–1935) began life as the son of a Scottish farmer and ended it as Baron Woolavington—businessman, entrepreneur, philanthropist and multimillionaire. Buchanan was an astute businessman, an opportunist and a risk taker—some of the key characteristics that defined the ideals of British imperial masculinity.

In 1879, Buchanan left his employment in the grain trade in Glasgow and moved to London to work for a whisky firm. By 1884, he had accumulated enough knowledge and contacts in the whisky trade to start his own business.[9] As the retail side of the business grew, Buchanan began a process of backward integration to control the entire whisky manufacturing process through the purchase and control of distillers and bottling plants and in 1903 the company was registered as a limited company.[10] Ronald Weir believes that the success of Buchanan's early business strategy was down to his determination to climb the social ladder and seek prestigious clients and outlets for his products.[11] Buchanan was adept at selling his whisky in desirable places and to influential people. He doggedly pursued contracts and quickly managed to get his blend of whisky sold in London hotels, theatres and other prominent drinking venues. As Spiller notes, the House of Commons contract in 1885 was a significant coup that highlights two key features of Buchanan's sales strategy: one was exploiting opportunities and the second was promoting the brand.[12]

The 1890 Select Committee on British and Foreign Spirits asked an analytical chemist, Dr Bell, to test the whisky sold in the Houses of Parliament which was, of course, Buchanan's blend (see Appendix for more detail on Dr Bell's whisky test). This whisky test was seemingly conducted in order to aid the committee's deliberations over the correct labelling of spirits and to establish if products should state the country of origin. The Committee was particularly keen to gather scientific data and opinions on the differences between blended whiskies and malt whiskies, and on the purity and strength of whisky and other spirits. The House of Commons whisky brand fared well from Dr Bell's chemical analysis and Buchanan wasted no time in promoting the Committee's findings through bottle labelling (see Figs. 7.1, 7.2, and 7.3) Buchanan used bottle labelling as the chief way to cultivate an elite status for his brands of whisky and no opportunity was missed to convince people that Buchanan's whisky was the favoured drink of the social elites.

Buchanan secured royal warrants from Queen Victoria in 1898 and further royal warrants followed in 1901 from Edward VII and in 1910 from George V. This led to the marketing of the 'Royal Household' brand of whiskies which filled the gap left when the decision was taken in 1904 to officially change the 'House of Commons' brand to 'Black and White'. Although the supply to the House of Commons still appeared on labelling after this date, it was less blatant until it was finally removed in 1915. In most historical accounts the reason given for this change is

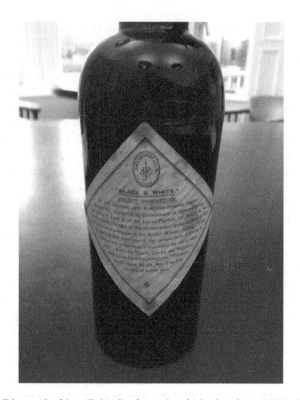

Fig. 7.1   Diageo Archive (DA): Buchanan's whisky bottle c. 1905, Courtesy of Diageo PLC[13]

that due to the design of the bottle customers began asking for 'that black and white whisky' (see Fig. 7.1). This suggests that the company were responsive to consumer feedback and demands and were therefore willing to cast aside social emulation in favour of more straightforward marketing tactics. This may have been true but it is not the only reason why the House of Commons branding was eventually withdrawn. The records of the House of Commons Kitchen Committee in conjunction with Buchanan's personal correspondence reveal the controversial nature of the company's marketing strategy and the determination to pursue it.

When Buchanan secured the contract to supply the Houses of Parliament in 1885 he saw the advertising potential of this deal. The words 'as specially selected for the House of Commons' appeared along

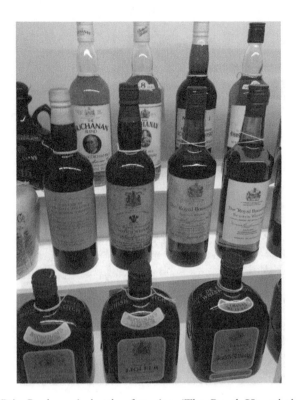

Fig. 7.2 DA: Buchanan's bottles featuring 'The Royal Household' labels c. 1910, Courtesy of Diageo PLC

with pictures of the Houses of Parliament on the labels of Buchanan's blended whiskies. Companies that supplied goods to the royal family also used this style of advertising on their products and therefore it must have seemed logical to promote the contract with the Houses of Parliament. However, the House of Commons Kitchen Committee which was responsible for the purchase and sale of alcoholic drinks within Parliament appeared to take exception to Buchanan's marketing tactics and in 1895 the order to supply whisky went to another firm. In November 1895 Buchanan wrote a letter to W. Tudor Howell MP, an acquaintance who had recently been elected to parliament, complaining that his contract to supply whisky to the House of Commons had not been renewed

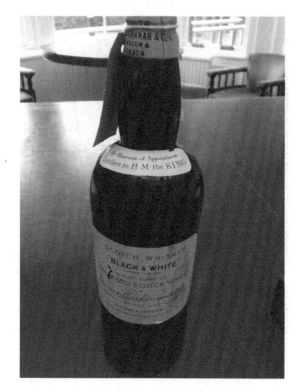

Fig. 7.3   DA: Buchanan's black and white whisky bottle c. 1910 labeled 'by warrant of appointment distillers to H. M. The King', Courtesy of Diageo PLC

I supplied Messrs.' Alexander Gordon & Co. Refreshment Contractors to the House of Commons with Scotch whisky, from December 1885 until the time when the House took the Refreshment Department under its own control. After this I continued to supply Scotch Whisky to the House and in December 1886, I was officially notified by the Kitchen Committee, that I was appointed supplier of Scotch Whisky to the Kitchen Department. Indeed, up to April 1893, I had practically the entire sup- ply in my hands. Never at any time was there complaint ... At the open- ing of the House in February 1893, I did not receive the customary order to supply. I called upon Mr Saunders, the Caterer, to ascertain the cause of this, as there had not been one word of complaint and no communi- cation of any kind from the Committee. Mr Saunders informed me that

the Committee had expressed displeasure at my making use, as an advertisement, of the fact that I supplied the House of Commons with Scotch
Whisky.[14]

The letter went on to say that Buchanan believed that he had 'only done
what any other firm would do' and used the examples of firms advertising the supply of goods to the royal household. He also pointed out that
his replacement (another whisky supplier Messrs.' Denman & Co.) were
now using the House of Commons supply as a form of advertisement on
bottles and business cards and he, therefore, felt that he had been particularly targeted

> But the great injustice to me is this. My whisky, which has all along been
> associated with the House of Commons, is understood by the public
> generally, and asked for as 'The House of Commons Blend'. The Trade
> now know that I do not supply the House, and this cessation of custom
> is doing me harm, as it is naturally assumed that my whisky has been
> dropped for good cause.[15]

Although there was no further correspondence to or from Mr Howell
about this matter, presumably the letter had some effect because by
1901 Buchanan was once again supplying the Houses of Parliament with
whisky. Labels on Buchanan Blend whisky from 1896 featured an extract
from a letter sent by the manager of the Refreshment Department in the
House of Commons, which confirmed that Buchanan had secured the
order to supply whisky to the department 'until further notice.'[16] Other
labels stated 'The Buchanan Blend, Special quality fine old Scotch whisky
as supplied to The House of Commons' or 'As supplied to The House
of Lords.'[17] So despite losing and then regaining the contract, Buchanan
calculated that the benefits of advertising outweighed the risks. The success of Buchanan Blend rested upon its reputation as an elite drink and
it was, therefore, vital to ensure continued consumer confidence in the
product.

The records of the Kitchen Committee reveal that they remained dis-
pleased with the use of the contract as a form of advertising. In the committee meetings of June 1901, there were discussions of sourcing other
whisky firms to fill the newly installed whisky vat.[18] However, in July, it
was resolved that the whisky vat should be filled 'on this occasion' with
Buchanan's blend and that Mr Buchanan should be informed that filling

the vat in the House of Commons should not be used as an advertisement.[19] Once again Buchanan chose to ignore this warning and carried on using the contract for advertising purposes. In 1905, the newly launched Black and White Blend labels included the statement 'Black and White specially selected for the House of Commons.'[20] Interestingly the Kitchen Committee, although clearly unhappy with the unwanted advertising, continued to order Buchanan's whisky. In March 1909, the committee once again discussed changing whisky suppliers but agreed to go with Buchanan. It is not clear from the records whether this was a financial decision or one based upon a preference for the whisky. In March 1912, it was again resolved to order Buchanan's whisky but noted that Mr Buchanan 'should be told to stop using this contract for advertising and trading purposes.'[21] However it took three years for Buchanan to take any notice and in 1915 all reference to the House of Commons was removed from labelling and from then on—until the 1990s in fact, the House of Commons brand was not sold to the general public but only within parliament. The timing of the move may have had something to do with the wartime restrictions on alcohol and it may have seemed inappropriate to draw attention to alcohol consumption within parliament. Yet Buchanan's reluctance to bend to the will of the Kitchen Committee any sooner is understandable: The company had staked its reputation on the supply of products to the highest institutions in the country and used advertising as a means of cultivating and promoting the idea that Scotch was a respectable drink. By 1915, these objectives had been achieved and therefore removing the House of Commons branding but maintaining the supply was a logical concession.

Buchanan & Co. invested time and money in formulating and implementing many other advertising strategies besides bottle labelling. By the turn of the century, the company was already a visible presence in London due to its delivery horse and carts, which were distinctive because all the horses were of the same breed, and were well trained and groomed. The drivers were smartly dressed and the vans were highly polished and clearly showed the Buchanan company name. By this time the company had developed a range of different whisky brands which varied in terms of price, age and strength. In 1897 Buchanan wrote to an old acquaintance in Kilmarnock, who was a master blender, to ask for advice on developing a cheaper brand of whisky 'I am anxious to get as successful a result as I can, and I am very desirous of getting the order, which will be large; but unfortunately it will be principally entirely a matter of price.'[22] In the 1890s when alcohol sales were falling, it was important to promote cheaper products in order to broaden and develop the domestic market. The company began using the trade press for advertising and between 1897 and 1898 adverts appeared in periodicals with a picture of Buchanan Blend along with a quote from *The Lancet* which stated 'Our analysis shows this to be a remarkably pure spirit and therefore well adapted for medicinally dietetic purposes'. The main advert heading stated 'Ordered by MPs and Doctors'. Adverts also appeared in illustrated weekly newspapers and provincial newspapers.[23]

Between 1904 and 1910 the subject of advertising was a constant theme raised at company board meetings. Buchanan sought to expand the business in England and Scotland and one of the most promising ways to do so was through the use of railway advertising and the sale of whisky in railway refreshment rooms, buffet cars and hotels. In September 1906, it was agreed that advertising show cards should be placed in North Eastern Railway refreshment rooms. It was resolved to increase advertising costs to one pound per show card per annum for not more than 30 show cards.[24] Over the next few years, the committee also agreed to place posters and show cards in the Midland, Great Northern Railway, London and South Western Railway, G&R and Bakerloo railway lines. It was proposed that the posters displayed in refreshment rooms and stations featured 'Morning Nip' advertisements, presumably encouraging consumers to drink Buchanan's whisky on the morning commute to work. Between 1908 and 1909 there were discussions of expanding advertising to the Eastern counties and Scotland and it was decided to place posters in the principle railway stations in Scotland and to accept advertising space at Glasgow Central Station for £100 per year. It was also agreed to place posters at various other Scottish railway stations and to pay 12 guineas to Highland Railway for stocking Buchanan's whisky for sale in buffet cars and in hotels. In addition, the committee agreed to advertise in Liverpool and surrounding stations to the total of 100 posters.[25]

Other advertising strategies were discussed such as theatre and hotel advertising but only certain 'high class' venues such as The Ritz hotel and The Lyric Theatre were deemed suitable. At one board meeting in February 1908, the subject of playing cards cropped up. The company had received letters from customers and others suggesting playing card advertising for the home trade but the suggestion was unanimously dismissed. This seems strange because the company had been reaching out to a broader range of consumers through newspaper and railway advertising, which suggests a strategy of selling products to consumers of all social classes but perhaps the association of playing cards with gambling was viewed as undesirable.

After 1910, the company developed the Black and White brand advertising which used the concept of 'black and white' to symbolise the ideals of British imperialism. The adverts initially featured two dogs: one a West Highland terrier and the other a Scottish terrier—one black and one white. The dogs had 'character' and breeding and they were distinctive because of their colours, which were contrasting and oppositional. Yet despite their differences the dogs always stood together, side by side, sometimes fighting a common enemy. For example, an advert from 1909 (Fig. 7.4) showed the two dogs sitting side by side with the caption 'Still Watchers' while another advert from 1910 featured the black and white dogs chained together chasing a rat and a cat.[26] The advertising also drew upon other 'black and white' themes such as the black and white women advert from 1909 (Fig. 7.5), which showed a 'black' woman walking behind a young 'white' woman in a manner suggesting a colonial mistress and maid relationship. Like the dog adverts, the concept of black and white represented a contrasting but seemingly complimentary relationship—there could not be one without the other; the white needed the black and vice versa; the colours represented a 'good blend' like the Scotch.

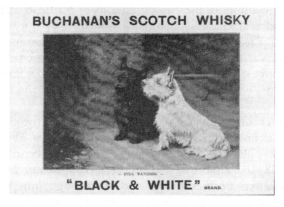

Fig. 7.4   DA: Buchanan's Black and White advert: 1909, Courtesy of Diageo PLC

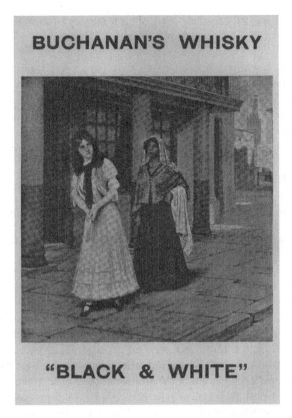

Fig. 7.5 DA: Buchanan's Black and White advert: 1909, Courtesy of Diageo PLC

Of course, Buchanan was not the only company to commodify British imperialism. An advert for Four Crown Scotch Whisky that appeared in the trade journal *The National Guardian* in September 1900 ran with the caption 'A Powerful Peacemaker' and showed a sketch of soldiers and prisoners in an army camp during the Boer War, sharing glasses of whisky. Beneath this scene the advert claimed

> While a prisoner of war in Pretoria, The Earl of Rosslyn, in a letter to the London *Daily Mail* of 11th July 1900 shows, how as soon as the news of Lord Roberts' approach reached the town almost everyone went wild with excitement. He says – "Hollander and Britisher, soldier and Boer peasant,

prisoner and warder, joined in a mutual expression of esteem and a glass of Robert Brown's Four Crown Scotch Whisky.

By 1900 Scotch was an imperial drink. Companies like Buchanan, Dewar and Walker had built up large export markets using imperial trade links. By this time Buchanan sold products in Australia, New Zealand, India, South Africa, Jamaica, South America, North Africa, Canada and the United States. An advert for Walker's whisky from 1910 showed an image of the famous 'Johnnie Walker striding man' with the caption

> Born in 1820 and still going strong – so when someone out in Calcutta or Borneo or Cape Town or Sydney or Valparaiso or any other little jaunt from 'home' laments that he cannot get the good old Scotch they have at 'home', call for Johnnie Walker, let him taste it, and tell him about the vast ageing reserve stock and the ninety years experience that make possible the guarantee.[27]

By 1910, Walker had developed the 'Johnnie Walker striding man' character, which was distinctive and resembled a rather (by that time) antiquated nineteenth-century upper-class dandy. In the adverts, the striding man was 'going strong since 1820' because this was the year when the company first began trading as a licensed grocer in Kilmarnock, Scotland. Like Buchanan, Walker also believed in the power of advertising and of creating a brand image that both promoted and reflected the ideals of British culture and imperialism. In the 1911 'Fashions come and go' campaign, the striding man was inserted into a variety of settings which depicted him as a gentlemanly protector. The adverts showed scenes of Johnnie Walker helping well-to-do ladies step over puddles; shielding them from rain and high winds and 'helping' ladies play a game of croquet.[28] These adverts drew upon concepts of class and gender in order to sell ideas about whisky to middle-class women who were the group most likely to buy Scotch from licensed grocers. The adverts promoted the idea that Johnnie Walker's whisky embodied the ideals of respectable masculinity—and therefore Scotch was a man's drink but it would certainly 'help' if ladies knew which brand to choose.

The success of companies like Buchanan and Walker lay in the ability to cultivate and expand the domestic and foreign markets for blended Scotch whisky. In Scotland, blended whisky was commonly drunk by the working classes because it was cheap and often bad—either watered down or adulterated with other intoxicants. The better quality blended 'Highland' whiskies were often produced in or around the central belt near Glasgow or Edinburgh and were subject to 'Scotch myths' marketing in order to boost sales. James Buchanan went further to completely reinvent blended whisky as a desirable and respectable drink of the British elites. His dogged pursuit of advertising via product labelling ensured that Buchanan whisky became firmly associated with ideas about quality, taste and privilege. The Johnnie Walker striding man is another example of product marketing designed to elevate the status of whisky and to Anglicise it—making it conceptually palatable for the English market. Both companies knew that the use value of whisky as an intoxicant held little currency compared to its cultural value and more specifically, it's potential as a source of cultural capital. Advertising played a key role in this process because it was vital to generate and maintain consumer interest, confidence and loyalty. The economic value of alcohol— in terms of expanding the drink trade and generating tax revenue—was largely dependent upon maintaining and developing the cultural value of the substance. If the cultural value evaporated amid a climate of temperance campaigning and legislative controls then there could be no market for alcohol. Therefore, the best way to keep people drinking was to sell them ideas about drinks that veered away from alcohol's primary effect of intoxication and instead promoted contemporary social values. However, as the Gilbey records show, by the turn of the century, maintaining the market for alcohol became more complex as consumers were increasingly drawn towards particular brands of alcoholic drinks that they associated with ideas about quality and taste.

NOTES

1. Townsend B. 2011. *Scotch Missed: Scotland's Lost Distilleries.* Glasgow: Neil Wilson Publishing Ltd: p. 31.
2. Spiller B. 1984. *The Chameleon's Eye: James Buchanan & Company Limited 1884–1984.* London and Glasgow: James Buchanan & Co. Ltd: p. 8.
3. Ibid.: p. 9.
4. Weir R. B. 1982. 'Distilling and Agriculture' in *Agricultural History Review:* pp. 49–62: www.bahs.org.uk/AGHR/ARTICLES/32nla4.pdf: accessed 4/11/2014.
5. Ibid.

6. Ibid.: p. 50.
7. Townsend B. 2011: p. 30.
8. 'James Buchanan's Obituary': *The Daily Express*: 27 August 1935.
9. Atherton F. W. 1931. *History of House Buchanan*: No Other Publication Details.
10. Weir R. B. 1974. 'The Distilling Industry in Scotland in the Nineteenth and Early Twentieth Centuries': PhD Dissertation: Edinburgh University: pp. 552–560.
11. Ibid.
12. Spiller B. 1984: p. 12.
13. The label on the bottle states: At the British and Foreign Spirits Select Committee appointed by the government in 1890, under the presidency of Lord Playfair, Dr Bell, CB, the chief analytical chemist of the government spoke in terms of high appreciation of a sample of our Scotch whisky saying 'From the general fine character of the sample there is reason to believe that it has been warehoused for many years etc.' Fifteen years later the Medical Magazine (October 1905) says the statement made by Dr Bell is as true today as it was then.
14. DA: Acc1033671: Buchanan's Letter Book: 1888–1897: Letter to W. Tudor Howell Esq MP: Dated 9 November 1895.
15. DA: Acc1033671: Buchanan's Letter Book: 1888–1897: Letter to W. Tudor Howell Esq MP: Dated 9 November 1895.
16. DA: Acc 125/3: Buchanan's Label Book: 1896.
17. DA: Acc 125/3: Buchanan's Label Book: 1896.
18. UK Parliamentary Archives (PA): House of Commons Kitchen Committee Records: HC/CL/CO/EA/2/2: Minute Books: 1901–1905.
19. Ibid.
20. DA: Acc 125/3: Buchanan's Label Book: 1905.
21. PA: House of Commons Kitchen Committee Records: HC/CL/CO/EA/2/3: 1906–1912.
22. DA: Letter Book: Acc103367/(1/2): 1897–1902: Letter from James Buchanan to David Sneddon: Dated 28 December 1897.
23. Spiller B. 1984: p. 34.
24. DA: Acc 100045/1: Buchanan Minute Books: 1906.
25. DA: Acc 100045/1: Buchanan Minute Books: 1906–1910.
26. DA: 884/43: Buchanan Black and White Adverts: 1910–1911.
27. DA: John Walker 'Striding Man' Advertising: 1908–1911.
28. DA: John Walker 'Striding Man' Advertising: 1908–1911.

CHAPTER 8

Selling the 'Illusion' of the Brand: W & A Gilbey

There are indeed many people who want to buy limited quantities of the best brandy than of the best champagne, as it is looked upon somewhat as a medicine that must be kept in the house, and it is just as difficult to get them to believe this can be obtained without the brand of Hennessey or Moet, as the finest champagne can be obtained under W&A Gilbey's Castle 4a or Castle 5a. We shall therefore, make just as large a profit on any goods we sell under these brands as if we sold them under the brand of W&A Gilbey, and shall thereby meet the wants and prejudices of two classes of consumers, and at the same time reap equal advantages both present and future out of either.[1]

W & A Gilbey began business in the wine and spirit trade in the 1850s as a family company run by three brothers, Walter, Alfred and Henry along with other male family members. The business expanded after the 1860 Licensing Act which led to the growth in the off-licence trade. The company appointed sales agents in most principle cities in Britain in order to stimulate and secure business with licensed grocers. Gilbey's interests lay principally in the retail side of the trade and the company bought wines and spirits which they either sold directly on to customers or bottled and labelled as their own brand of goods. However, as the quote above indicates, the demand for branded goods increased towards the end of the century and the company was forced to restructure its business model in order to meet customer demand and secure the market for its products.

© The Author(s) 2018
T. Hands, *Drinking in Victorian and Edwardian Britain*,
https://doi.org/10.1007/978-3-319-92964-4_8

The company produced a price list in 1896 that was designed to promote its market position as the leading retailer of wines and spirits. It claimed that during 1895 every 14th bottle of wine and every 35th bottle of spirits consumed in Britain had been sold by W & A Gilbey.[2] The price lists from 1870 to 1896 featured a broad range of wines, spirits and beers that were purchased and then rebranded under Gilbey's 'Castle' brand name. The Castle branding was given to a range of drinks, such as brandy, gin, whisky, sherry, port, liqueurs, champagnes and wines. The price lists were extensive and contained detailed information on the types of drinks, their origin, strength, qualities and uses. Although the Castle brand dominated the price lists, by 1890, sales agents reported complaints from customers who wanted particular brands of wine and spirits that Gilbey did not supply. The company was therefore forced to rethink its position on the supply of branded goods.

There was a realisation that in order to compete in a changing market for alcohol, the company would have to give customers what they wanted—which was the 'illusion' cast by particular brand names which conferred ideas about quality, taste and status. The committee agreed to expand the sale of branded goods and decided to deal with five prominent wine houses: Croft & Co., Silva & Cosens (Dow), Gonzales Byass & Co., Ingham Whitaker and Cossart Gordon & Co.[3] It was also agreed to provisionally deal with Burgoyne & Co. for the supply of Australian wines because it was noted that 'the introduction of Australian Wines has afforded us an insight of the power of certain brands over the public, and the additional customers that our agents have secured for them.'[4] The committee also discussed the purchase of wine that had been rebranded under the Castle label which simply listed the type of wine, for example sauvignon etc. It was noted that

It is a very fortunate thing for us that a knowledge of brands on the part of the public have only gone as far as champagne and brandy, which has naturally been owing to their having been bottled abroad, when the shippers have been enabled to place their name before the public rather than the wine merchant on this side. The reputation of champagne is entirely owing to the fact that the wine must be bottled in the place of production … It would however be impossible to make one name famous alike for ports, sherries, whiskies, brandies and W&A Gilbey never can hope to do so. They can, however, easily make themselves famous for supplying the finest brands of every country and it is important that they should lose no time in endeavouring to make the names of the Houses they have allied themselves with equally famous to the public as they now are to the trade before attempts are made to supply the public with other.[5]

By selling brands that would in essence compete with their own brand of goods, the company believed it would secure its position in the market because it could promote its own goods alongside others. In the 1860s, the company had entered into a contract with John Jameson & Sons to purchase large quantities of whisky from Jameson's Irish distillery. The whisky was held in bonded warehouses in Dublin and then marketed under the Gilbey brand name 'Castle Grand JJ'. This branding partnership had been successful in securing sales of Jameson's whisky until the 1890s when Scotch whisky captured the market position previously held by Irish whisky. By 1890, it was felt that rebranding Jameson's whisky would help boost sales and therefore all reference to W & A Gilbey was removed from the labelling. However, this clearly did not remedy the situation and in 1897 the committee produced a report, which included an interview with Jameson himself. The report stated that

> He [Jameson] referred to the decline in England in the consumption of Irish, compared with the great strides made in Scotch whisky. He remarked in a jocular way "we are not going to give up the game yet, but want to do all we can to popularise Dublin whisky in England, and we think you can help us."[6]

Jameson suggested that Gilbey's sales agents ask grocers to display show cards for JJ whisky alongside any adverts for Scotch. Jameson did not want to advertise his products in any other way and refused advertising in railway stations but preferred adverts in grocers at the point of sale. He was told that it was not within the company's power to compel customers to advertise Jameson's whisky. Jameson pointed out that their mutual arrangement and success depended on the continued trade in Irish whisky in England and that in Ireland he could 'run alone' but needed help to sell his goods in England.[7] However, the committee felt that they could only go so far in promoting Jameson's whisky and if sales in Irish whisky in England were declining then the company's focus should instead be placed on the marketing of Scotch.

Rebranding Castle Grand JJ had not halted declining sales in Irish whisky but the committee still believed that removing the W & A Gilbey name from Jameson's whisky and their own Glen Spey Scotch would improve brand confidence. The 1897 committee report effectively recommended the removal of the Gilbey name from all but the cheapest brands.[8] The logic for this was based on an analysis of sales which identified four types of consumers: First, there were those who wanted to buy the cheapest products if they were known to be genuine; Second were those who wanted a 'fair medium price article.'; Third were consumers who wanted the finest quality products regardless of name or brand; Fourth were those who wanted the best brand regardless of quality. The report went on to state that

> The public cannot be brought to feel that W&A Gilbey with all their advantages of wealth and commercial knowledge which they give them credit for, possess the same opportunities of buying ports and sherries or Marsala and Madeiras as Croft and Dow or Gonzales, Crossart and Ingham. They imagine these brands are connected with the production of certain favoured vineyards and form monopolies of these Houses ... If during the last few years we have increased our reputation for selling pure but cheap wine, we have also considerably increased our commercial reputation and the public are disposed to place unbounded confidence in us when we state that Croft's Port and Gonzales Sherry are the finest, but are very loathe to believe us when we endeavour to crack open our own goods such as Castle J Port and Castle A Sherry, no matter what the quality may be. ... The whole of our success is to be traced to names, brands, vintages etc. which by degrees we have added to our price list.[9]

From the analysis of consumers and based on the information from sales agents, the company had decided that the Castle label could only fill a certain niche in the market. By the turn of the century, consumers wanted branded goods and therefore the company focus had to shift accordingly. When the business had taken off in the 1860s, Gilbey's customers were less 'brand driven' and were content to buy many products from reputable wine and spirit merchants. By the turn of the century however, the company name and reputation could no longer be relied upon to generate sufficient alcohol sales because unbranded products could not be consumed conspicuously. Brand names of particular types of alcoholic drinks were well known—even the more expensive ones and sometimes the form of advertising was particularly innovative.

A good example of this was found in the music halls which emerged in the second half of the nineteenth century from pubs that offered entertainments.[10] These places ranged from small 'penny gaffs' located in pubs to large venues such as theatres.[11] By the turn of the century, music halls had grown in popularity by offering cheap entertainment to the urban working classes in cities across Britain.[12] One of the most popular acts in the late Victorian period was a musical pastiche of upper-class men known as the 'swell song'. Bailey describes a swell as 'a lordly figure of resplendent dress and confident air whose exploits centered on drink and women.'[13] The most famous (or indeed infamous) performer of the swell song was George Leybourne with his act 'Champagne Charlie'. Leybourne's theatrical success was built upon his sharp observations of the drinking habits of the rich, which was wrung out for a laugh to the appreciation of the music hall crowds. Leybourne wrote the lyrics for Champagne Charlie

> The way I gained my title's
> By a hobby which I've got
> Of never letting others pay
> However long the shot
> Whoever drinks at my expense
> Are treated all the same
> From Dukes to Lords to cabmen down
> I make them drink champagne
>
> From coffee and from supper rooms
> From Poplar to Pall Mall
> The girls on seeing me exclaim
> "Oh what a champagne swell"!
> The notion 'tis of everyone
> If 'twere not for my name
> And causing so much to be drunk
> They'd never make champagne
>
> Some epicures like Burgundy,
> Hock, Claret and Moselle,
> But Moet' s vintage only
> Satisfies this champagne swell
> What matters if to bed I go
> Dull head and muddled thick
> A bottle in the morning
> Sets me right then very quick

Chorus
For Champagne Charlie is my name
Champagne Charlie is my game
Good for any game at night, my boys
Good for any game at night, my boys
For Champagne Charlie is my name
Champagne Charlie is my game
Good for any game at night, my boys
Who'll come and join me in the spree?[14]

The idea that Champagne Charlie kept the champagne industry in business through his prolific drinking bore some reality to the free supply of champagne gifted to Leybourne from London wine merchants in return for publicity.[15] So it would seem that the reference to Moet was perhaps intentional. Although there is no evidence to suggest that Gilbey & Co. supplied champagne to Leybourne or any other music hall performer, the Champagne Charlie act demonstrates the ways in which ideas about particular brands of alcoholic drinks were propagated.

In the consumer society that emerged in the late nineteenth century, Veblen's ideas about conspicuous consumption were evident. The Gilbey records show that customers were increasingly brand-driven, demanding particular types of wines, spirits and champagnes that could be consumed as markers of wealth, status or taste. The company knew that it was impossible to convince customers that its own-brand products were of an equal quality and therefore relegated only the cheapest products to the company branding. This in turn elevated the status of branded goods to those which were more expensive and therefore all the more exclusive and desirable. In this sense, the 'illusion' of the brand was a powerful and persuasive way to secure the market for alcohol.

NOTES

1. Diageo Archives (DA): 100433/1: W & A Gilbey Committee Minutes: 1890.
2. DA: 100422/190: W & A Gilbey Price Lists: 1870–1896.
3. Ibid.
4. DA: 100433/1: W & A Gilbey Committee Minutes: 1890.
5. DA: 100433/1: W & A Gilbey Committee Minutes: 1890.
6. DA: 100433/1: W & A Gilbey Committee Minutes: 1897.
7. DA: 100433/1: W & A Gilbey Committee Minutes: 1897.

8. DA: 100433/1: W & A Gilbey Committee Minutes: 1897.
9. DA: 100433/1: W & A Gilbey Committee Minutes: 1897.
10. Maloney P. 1993. *Scotland and the Music Hall 1850–1914*: Manchester: Manchester University Press: pp. 24–57.
11. Bailey P. 2003. *Popular Culture and Performance in the Victorian City*. Cambridge: Cambridge University Press: p. 100.
12. Maloney: pp. 24–57.
13. Bailey: p. 101.
14. Ibid.: pp. 109–110.
15. Ibid.

PART III

Drinking in Victorian and Edwardian Britain

The final part contains four chapters that offer different and sometimes contrasting perspectives on the reasons why alcohol was consumed and on the drinking cultures that emerged from the Victorian period. Alcohol played a key role in the everyday lives of men and women across Britain. It was not only consumed in pubs, restaurants, theatres, refreshment rooms and many other public places but also in the privacy of people's homes or in private members clubs. People drank for many different reasons and these reasons ranged across social class, gender and region. In the nineteenth century, alcohol still held a vital place in medical practice and was prescribed for a range of physiological and psychological illnesses. Even when its use in therapeutics began to fall out of fashion, late Victorian consumers relied upon alcohol as a tonic that could be used for the purposes of self-medication.

CHAPTER 9

Doctor's Orders: A Prescription to Drink

During the last few years there has been a decided boom in certain sophisticated wines – 'dietetic' or 'tonic' or 'restorative' beverages. Undoubtedly the public imagination has been captured by the ingenious methods pursued in pushing these productions ... [Of] those most puffed in the newspapers and advertised in the press and on public boardings, it may be safely affirmed that they have no appreciable therapeutic influence other than that possessed by any of the ordinary wines on the market.[1]

Throughout the Victorian and Edwardian periods, people consumed alcohol for health reasons. This was driven in part by the use of alcohol in medical practice and also by commercial factors, which played a significant role in promoting ideas about the health benefits of consuming certain alcoholic drinks. The quote above is from an article on the sale of tonic wines in the *British Journal of Inebriety* in 1910. The article offered a scathing attack on what the writer referred to as the 'ingenious' and 'aggressive' marketing of tonic wines which were accused of holding little therapeutic value and could potentially lead to alcoholism.[2] The writer, a doctor and magistrate, noted the popularity of tonic wines which were one of many types of proprietary remedies widely available in the late Victorian period. This chapter explores the issue of drinking for health in the late Victorian and early Edwardian periods by examining the controversy that surrounded the medicinal use of alcohol. Debates about the efficacy of alcohol as a therapeutic agent circulated in medical journals towards the end of the century. An analysis of hospital records

© The Author(s) 2018
T. Hands, *Drinking in Victorian and Edwardian Britain*,
https://doi.org/10.1007/978-3-319-92964-4_9

shows that although its usage diminished in the period leading up to the First World War, doctors still relied upon it to treat a range of physiological and psychological illnesses. Alcohol had been used as a staple drug in medical practice since the seventeenth century.[3] Its usage within medicine continued throughout the nineteenth and twentieth centuries and the general public therefore had good reason to believe in its medicinal power. Prescriptions for alcohol became increasingly popular in the nineteenth century when more heroic methods of treatment such as cupping and bloodletting fell out of use. However, doctors came under attack from temperance campaigners both inside and outside of the medical profession because a prescription to drink had moral and medical implications and by the end of the century, its usage within hospitals and asylums had declined.

By the late nineteenth century, debates existed on the therapeutic value of alcohol and despite its enduring status as a staple medicine, some doctors avoided prescribing it altogether. At the core of these debates was the issue of therapeutic nihilism—whether prescribing alcohol actually did more harm than good. The effects of alcohol on health were poorly understood and medical opinions were not only based on scientific evidence but sometimes on moral grounds. In a presidential address given to the British Society for the Study of Inebriety in July 1907, Dr Harry Campbell scrutinised the contents of a recently published medical manifesto on the influence of alcohol on health. He focused on a section of the manifesto which claimed that in the opinion of the medical signatories moderate drinking was beneficial to health

It is [according to the manifesto] the "moderate" use of alcoholic beverages that is held to be "usually beneficial." Now, what are we to understand by moderate? The signatories make no attempt to define the word. They should have told us what they regard as the limits of moderation - how much, i.e., a person may drink daily without forfeiting the claim to be considered a moderate drinker. Is moderate indulgence the equivalent of one, two, three, or four glasses of whisky per diem? Are we to take as the standard of moderation, the smallest or the largest quantity of alcohol daily consumed by any one of the signatories, or the mean of their respective total daily consumption? We need explicit information on this head. The term "moderate" is in truth a highly elastic one, possessing very different meanings for different individuals. I recently asked a casual acquaintance what he understood by moderate and he gave as answer "half a bottle of whisky a day." And I told him that I was going to suggest two glasses, or their equivalent to which he replied that a man who limited himself to so small a quantity was to all intents and purposes a teetotaller![4]

Campbell went further to suggest that the failure to quantify moderate drinking was matched by a failure to stipulate which types of alcohol should be considered 'moderate drinks' that were beneficial to health. He believed that the quality and type of alcohol were key factors in determining its effects on human health. Campbell concluded that

> The mouthpiece of the British medical profession, would have you to understand that nine-tenths of you will be benefited in health by the moderate use of alcoholic beverages, but we leave it to you to decide what a moderate quantity is, and you may choose any kind of alcoholic drink your fancy prompts.[5]

Doctors could not agree on 'healthy' amounts of alcohol consumption or if alcohol was beneficial in therapeutics. In a presidential address to The British Medical Association in 1905, Dr James Barr gave a speech on the use of alcohol as a therapeutic agent in which he argued that less alcohol was prescribed because of 'fashion' rather than from any scientific reasoning on its usefulness as a medicine

> There is no other drug in the pharmacopeia that has such an accommodating action to circumstances. It would seem as if in any particular case we could never predicate as to whether alcohol is going to do good or harm. Surely some indications could be laid down for its use so that we should know beforehand what effect it is going to produce.[6]

Barr called for more scientific research on the uses and effects of alcohol as a therapeutic drug because he believed that it remained useful in medicine and more importantly, despite the controversy over its use, many doctors still prescribed it anyway. To illustrate this point Barr set out the principal therapeutic uses of alcohol in treating a range of illnesses: In the treatment of pneumonia he personally recommended the use of a 'light draught beer' as a sedative and in typhoid fever a 'pint of good bitter' was given in small doses over twenty-four hours. Cases of vomiting were treated with small doses of champagne and brandy was administered in cases of collapse or shock. For palliative care, he noted that diluted brandy was often given freely in the last days of life and for invalids it was common to prescribe 'a good port' during periods of convalescence.[7] In the treatment of nervous diseases, alcohol was used as a sedative and an analgesic. Cases of neuralgia were treated with a 'glass of good stout' and for cases of angina, hot whisky or brandy were recommended.[8] Barr described alcohol as a versatile drug that was available in a variety of forms that could be used to treat a range of illnesses. He believed that this made it a valuable medicine that should not be swept aside by fashion or moral concerns. Yet some doctors were critical of what they believed to be the morally questionable practice of prescribing alcohol. In 1885, Dr Norman Kerr, the prominent temperance campaigner and founder of the British Society for the Study of Inebriety, urged caution when prescribing any alcohol

> We can never forget that intoxicating drinks cannot be ordered without some risk of a taste for them being acquired, and the remedy itself proving worse than the original disease. This risk was exemplified in the case of a favourite dog of two maiden ladies of my acquaintance. This animal was seized with an attack of acute pneumonia. The veterinary surgeon gave the dog brandy; and the dog recovered, whether because of or in spite of the stimulant, I cannot tell. Ever since, if he hears anyone speak of brandy, he is up in a moment on his hind legs, begging for the seductive physic. Though I believe the cases of what may be called 'medical drunkenness' are not nearly as numerous as is popularly asserted, I have known instances where the medical prescription of strong drinks has been the beginning of a career of excess.[9]

Kerr's opinion was based on his belief that for some individuals (and dogs), alcohol was a dangerously addictive substance. He, therefore, believed that the continued use of alcohol in therapeutics could lead to an increase in cases of 'medical drunkenness' which could in turn damage the reputation of the profession. In a speech given two decades later to the Lancashire and Cheshire branch of the British Medical Profession, Dr Charles Macfie echoed Kerr's views regarding the use of alcohol in medicine.[10] Macfie believed that doctors had a duty to promote and support temperance reform, particularly when increasing scientific evidence and medical opinions suggested that alcohol was not conducive to good health. Like Kerr, he also believed that by continuing to prescribe alcohol, the medical profession risked damaging its reputation. Macfie gave the example of recent accusations by some temperance groups that increasing amounts of inebriety were due to taking alcohol 'under doctor's orders'

> This insinuation is a glaring economy of the truth and before such insinuations are published to the world, one would expect any fair minded society or individual to first probe the truth about 'doctor's orders.' There are two sides to a ladder. No drunkard ever takes the blame for his or her degraded condition as the profession so well knows. According to them, their own family circle and nearest friends are their direst enemies; and how often has a chimerical 'doctor's order' been given as an excuse! I could understand our being urgently requested to avoid prescribing alcohol in any form, on account of the moderate use of it becoming a habit and ultimately developing into a craving. The medical profession is as anxious that alcohol should not be abused and that human beings should not suffer in mind and body from its effects, as any teetotaller can possibly be.[11]

Although he had reservations about the validity of the claims made by the temperance groups, Macfie remained concerned that prescribing alcohol could bring the profession into disrepute because a prescription to drink could be risky—not only in terms of ethics but also in the damage it might do to professional reputation. Yet others were concerned about the implications of reducing or stopping the use of alcohol in medicine. In an article in the *British Medical Journal* in 1890, one doctor (who remained anonymous) highlighted the differences in alcohol use between workhouses and general hospitals

> The general hospitals throughout the country have very materially reduced their expenditure on alcohol in all its forms, but the general hospitals have not abandoned its use *in toto* ... The class of cases in the union infirmaries [where no alcohol was prescribed] are exactly identical with those in the general hospitals. The workhouse medical officer has to treat pneumonia and other acute diseases and grave surgical operations are performed in many union hospitals. At the Leeds General Infirmary alcohol is used. Must we conclude that the staff of Leeds General Infirmary are wrong in continuing this agent?[12]

Evidently, this doctor was concerned that the welfare of patients was put at risk by a distinction based on moral rather than medical grounds. Alcohol still held value within therapeutics and in surgical procedures and therefore to deny it to patients within workhouse hospitals must have seemed ethically questionable. However, temperance debates aside, by the early twentieth century there was growing scientific evidence for restricting the use of alcohol in medicine. Macfie referred to several studies that challenged the prevailing view that alcohol provided stimulation in cases of disease and debility.[13] These studies showed that alcohol also had an irritant or depressive action on nerves and body tissues. Macfie also pointed out that there were alternatives to alcoholic stimulation in therapeutics

> In turning to our *Pharmacopeia* and our *Extra Pharmacopeia* for substitutes for alcohol, we are at once impressed with the fact that most drugs have more or less stimulant properties, either local or general, for example, phosphorus, arsenic and iron, chloroform and the ethers, and the various alkaloids – all stimulant in medicinal doses.[14]

By the early twentieth century, there were pharmaceutical alternatives to alcohol that challenged its efficacy as a drug. Yet some doctors still believed that alcohol had an important place within therapeutics. In a speech given in 1909 to the Border Counties Branch of the British Medical Profession, Dr James MacDonald set out a convincing argument in favour of the continued, judicious use of alcohol in the treatment of illness and disease.[15] He argued that advances in medical knowledge were not sufficient to dismiss the role of alcohol as a valuable medicine

> There are of course habits and fashions in therapeutics as in everything else. Fashions in the past have sometimes been regulated by the prevailing theory of the origin of disease. In the days, for example, when diseases were set down to inflammation, bloodletting was all the vogue, and the use of alcohol was looked on as a perilous enormity. Then came the period when our bodily ills were ascribed to lowered vitality, and the stimulants were administered to therapeutic excess. At the present day, the bacterial origin of disease does not materially affect the employment of alcohol, which is generally given with judgment and discretion.[16]

In other words, the advent of germ theory did not radically change the role of alcohol in therapeutics. MacDonald believed that increased knowledge of the aetiology of disease meant that alcohol was prescribed more accurately and only when absolutely necessary. He argued that this change was not enough for the medical advocates of temperance reform who warned the profession to stop prescribing alcohol or face 'the high

road to therapeutic nihilism.'[17] Which meant that by continuing to prescribe alcohol the medical profession risked doing more harm than good.
MacDonald questioned the professional integrity of medical men who
put their 'extreme' personal beliefs about temperance above their duty to
patients. He cited an article published in *The Lancet* in 1908 written by a
group of 'well-known medical experts' who expressed the view that alcohol was a 'rapid and trustworthy restorative' that in some cases could be
a 'life saving drug.'[18] MacDonald believed that the majority of doctors
shared these views

> The manifesto discharges a kindly service as a protest against the uncom-
> promising opposition of a body of extremists to the rational use of alcohol.
> It does more – it applies a spur to the indifference displayed by many med-
> ical men with regard to an eminently practical question. It is true that on
> minor points a divergence of opinion exists, but on fundamental principles
> there is common agreement.[19]

This 'common agreement' was evident in hospital records which show
that up until the First World War alcohol was still used in large urban
voluntary hospitals and asylums. Although its use may have courted controversy among medical men and temperance organisations, the continued use of alcohol indicates that it was still widely regarded as a reliable
therapeutic drug. There were very few prescription drugs that offered
the same degree of versatility to treat fevers, disease, debility and provide
a degree of comfort for patients during the course of illness. Alcohol was
the rational drug of choice because it was relatively cheap, widely available and came in a variety of different forms that suited the needs of a
wide range of patients.

ALCOHOL USE IN HOSPITALS AND ASYLUMS

The value of alcohol was evident in hospital records which show that various types of alcoholic drinks were used in the treatment of patients suffering from a range of psychological and physiological conditions. The
records of four Glasgow hospitals show that between 1870 and 1914,
alcohol was still used in the treatment of patients. During this period,
Glasgow was one of the largest industrial cities in Britain and rapid population growth meant increasing problems associated with ill health and
disease.[20] The city therefore makes a good case study for the therapeutic

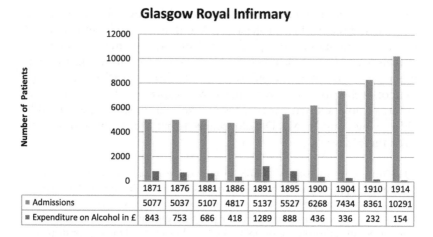

Graph 9.1   Glasgow Royal Infirmary alcohol expenditure from 1871 to 1914. The dates shown are those in which expenditure on alcohol was listed in the annual reports[21]

use of alcohol in the treatment of illness. The records of Glasgow Royal Infirmary; Gartnavel Royal Lunatic Asylum; The Western Infirmary and Hawkhead Asylum show increasing numbers of admissions in the late Victorian and Edwardian periods. Hospital expenditure on alcohol sometimes correlated with the number of admissions either increasing or decreasing according to the numbers of patients admitted and treated. Yet as the graphs show, between 1875 and 1914 there was a general trend towards growing numbers of admissions and decreasing expenditure on alcohol (Graph 9.1).

The graph shows that until 1895 alcohol use fluctuated. In 1891 there was a sharp increase in expenditure on alcohol but it is unclear from the records why more was spent in that year. It could be that particular types of admissions required treatment with alcohol. According to the 1891 records of the Registrar General for Scotland the highest numbers of deaths in Glasgow in that year were from bronchitis and pneumonia, which were predominantly secondary infections. The highest numbers of deaths from contagious diseases in 1891 related to measles, whooping cough and phthisis (tuberculosis).[22] It may be that these types of illnesses required therapeutic treatment with alcoholic stimulants. The

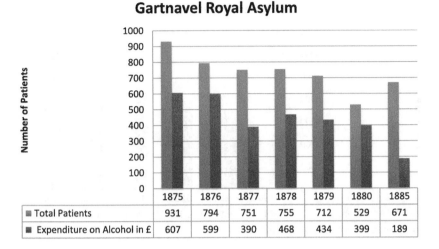

Gartnavel Royal Asylum

	1875	1876	1877	1878	1879	1880	1885
Total Patients	931	794	751	755	712	529	671
Expenditure on Alcohol in £	607	599	390	468	434	399	189

Graph 9.2   Gartnavel Royal Asylum alcohol expenditure from 1875 to 1885. The dates shown are those in which alcohol expenditure was listed in the annual reports[23]

graph shows that by 1914, despite a large amount of civilian and military admissions, the use of alcohol had declined. The wartime restrictions on alcohol may account in part for this decrease (Graph 9.2).

The graph shows fluctuating levels of expenditure on alcohol until 1879 when there was a marked trend towards higher admissions and less spent on alcohol. There is no evidence in the annual reports of decisions taken to restrict the medicinal use of alcohol but the increased numbers of admissions in 1885 coupled with the decreased expenditure on alcohol suggest a shift in hospital policy (Graph 9.3).

The data from the Western Infirmary shows a negative correlation between increasing numbers of admissions from 1895 onwards and decreasing expenditure on alcohol. By 1905, alcohol expenditure had fallen significantly despite a sharp increase in admissions in the same year. This is a similar pattern to that found in Glasgow Royal Infirmary and may be indicative of the financial constraints posed by larger numbers of admissions. This contrasts with the data shown below from a smaller institution, Hawkhead asylum where expenditure on alcohol remained fairly consistent until 1912 when it began to decline (Graph 9.4).

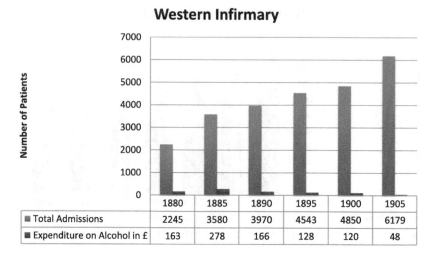

Graph 9.3 Western Infirmary alcohol expenditure from 1880 to 1905. The dates were selected at five-year intervals[24]

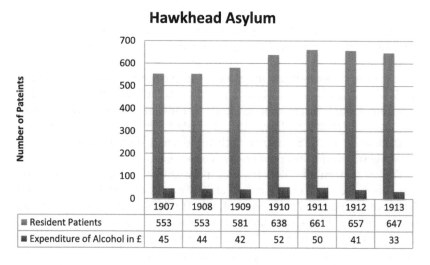

Graph 9.4 Alcohol expenditure in Hawkhead Asylum 1907–1913. The dates shown are those in which expenditure on alcohol was listed in the annual reports[25]

The data from the Glasgow hospitals suggests that overall expenditure on alcohol varied across different types of institutions and changed over time. It also shows a general trend towards restricting expenditure on alcohol. It is however difficult to ascertain exactly how the alcohol purchased was used in the treatment of patients and why this changed over time. In each of the institutions, the ward casebooks and patient notes lacked detailed information on treatment regimes and more specifically, on any alcohol prescribed. There was a case in Gartnavel Royal Asylum of a male patient admitted in 1888 suffering from 'low mood' exacerbated by bronchitis, who was prescribed 4 grams of whisky daily plus an expectorant mixture.[26] In the annual report for 1871, the medical superintendent of Gartnavel discussed the use of alcohol and stated that

> There are a number of weak, helpless bed-rid patients, especially in the East House, suffering from various diseases of long standing, many of whom were organically affected on admission ... While all the patients require to be well nourished and supported and are so, these patients, in consequence of their greater want of vitality, often require food to be expressly prepared for them and with stimulants to be administered both night and day with a large amount of kind and considerate treatment.[27]

It would therefore appear that alcohol played an important role in the treatment of chronic diseases and palliative care. In another Scottish asylum, The Chrichton Royal, alcohol was sometimes used in the treatment of private patients—even those with existing alcohol problems. One patient admitted in 1886 suffering from eccentric and delusional behaviour was allowed generous amounts of alcohol. His case notes stated that

> Mr H has resided at Kirkmichael House all winter and has had shooting all the season. He has been fairly contented as long as he had unlimited meal and drink. His appetite was enormous and at a meal he has been known to eat a leg of mutton with the usual accessories...and finish off with half a dozen eggs...he has been allowed three glasses of whisky daily and as much beer as he chose to drink. He usually took the whisky undiluted.[28]

This case highlights the differences in treatment with alcohol among private and pauper patients. Even if viewed as a necessary therapeutic agent, alcohol was an additional expense in the course of treatment and perhaps one that hospitals with larger numbers of pauper patients could ill afford.

In addition to the asylums, alcohol was also used in the treatment of infectious diseases in Belvedere (fever) Hospital in Glasgow. In the 1866 annual report the medical superintendent of Belvedere noted that during the typhus epidemic of 1861 and 1862, the hospital admitted 1837 patients and of these, 1289 were typhus cases.[29] The alcohol consumed during this period was: 62,754 ounces of wine, 8440 ounces of whisky and 2611 ounces of brandy.[30] The Medical Superintendent, Dr Russell believed that it was important to weigh up the therapeutic benefits of 'alcoholic stimulation' with the economic considerations. He stated that during the typhus epidemic, Belvedere Hospital and Glasgow Royal Infirmary had admitted similar numbers of typhus cases and that both hospitals had used alcohol in the treatment of patients. Yet Belvedere had successfully treated patients with a more judicious use of alcoholic stimulants than the Royal Infirmary. In fact, Dr Russell claimed that there were fewer deaths from typhus in Belvedere than in the Royal Infirmary and that the average length of stay was considerably less in the former.[31]

The use of alcohol in treating fevers and other illnesses was reported in medical journals. Aside from the financial implications of alcohol use, some doctors believed that it only held therapeutic value in certain cases and in particular stages of illness and disease. In an article in the *British Medical Journal* in 1880, Dr H. McNaughton a physician in The Fever Hospital Cork, provided evidence to support his claim that alcohol should be prescribed carefully in fever cases.[32] He kept records of his patients from January 1873 to June 1879, a period in which he treated 889 fever cases mainly typhus, typhoid and simple fever. On average 30% of patients were treated with alcohol during this period.[33] Most fever cases were treated using brandy, claret and wine. He provided a patient case study of a girl he described as being one of the worst cases of typhoid fever he had ever treated. In the early stages of her illness he prescribed no alcohol but instead treated her using milk, beef extract, foulbroth, digitalis, ipecacuanha (an expectorant sometimes used to treat dysentery), Dover's Powders, quinine and opium. In the later stages of illness, he prescribed a mixture of brandy and milk every four hours and one ounce of claret every two hours. The girl recovered completely.[34]

The type of alcohol used in the treatment of illness and disease varied. This was reflected in the Glasgow hospital data. The most popular types of alcohol purchased during the 1870–1914 period were wines and champagne, brandy, whisky, porter and beer. Most hospitals held

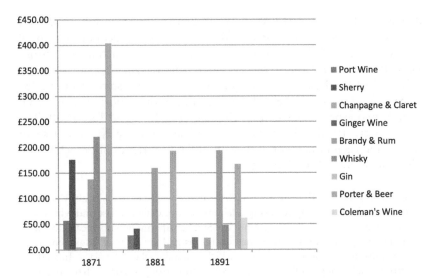

Graph 9.5 Types of alcohol purchased by Glasgow Royal Infirmary 1871–1891[35]

accounts with local wine and spirit merchants and the Royal Infirmary bought alcohol from two Glasgow firms: Samuel Dow and Thomas Anderson. The quantities and types of drinks purchased changed from year to year, sometimes reflecting the numbers of patients treated but at other times it seemed that certain drinks became more popular or fell out of use. Graph 9.5 shows the changing types and quantities of alcohol purchased by Glasgow Royal Infirmary over a 30-year period.

Certain types of drinks like porter and port wine remained popular over the 30-year period. Sherry fell out of use but champagne and claret were in more demand towards the end of the century. Coleman's Wincarnis Tonic Wine was purchased for the first time in 1891 with a sizeable order totalling £61 3s 12d, which in today's money equates to an annual spend of around £3665 on tonic wine.[36] The data from the Glasgow hospitals suggests that between 1870 and 1914, the types of alcohol purchased by hospitals changed, and that although there was an overall trend towards spending less on alcohol, its usage continued.

As many doctors still prescribed alcohol, it fell to the medical profession to investigate its role in the treatment of illness and disease.

Between 1880 and 1914 there were articles in *The British Medical Journal* and *The Lancet* that investigated the use of alcohol in medical practice. Some of these articles provided chemical analyses of various alcoholic drinks because it was considered important that doctors were informed of the best types and quality of wines and spirits to prescribe to patients. Following the reduction in duties on imported wines from France, two articles appeared in *The Lancet* in June and July 1880. The articles were titled 'The Lancet Commission on the Medical Use of Wines' and each instalment dealt with different varieties of French wines. The first article in June 1880 stated

> We cannot believe that any wines whatever are necessary for a healthy adult in good physical strength, taking a fair amount of daily exercise and with no excessive mental strain. Most light wines taken sparingly with meals do no harm to a person under the same conditions and are quite as consistent as the consumption of tea, coffee etc. which generally take their place. Indeed, strong tea, strong coffee and (we would add strong tobacco) have much to answer for in the production of indigestion and nervous palpitation ... To the invalid, the wines are frequently of great value and in some of the acute fevers the most powerful alcoholic beverages have sometimes to be prescribed ... [However] the patient's daily question "what shall I drink?" requires more consideration than is usually devoted to it before the medical advisor gives the stereotyped reply "Oh you can take a little claret".[37]

Both articles aimed to educate doctors on the composition and therapeutic value of various types of French wines. This was achieved by providing chemical analyses of the four basic constituents of wines, namely alcohol, sugar, acid and tannin. The articles claimed that differing levels of each of these constituents not only altered the taste and quality of the wine but also its therapeutic value.[38] In the case of claret it was noted that there were huge differences in the quality and chemical composition of this particular type of wine but it was still believed to have medicinal applications

> In cases of anaemia, ordinary debility from overwork, feeble digestion etc., a sound red claret is almost as good a prescription as most of the tonic drugs in the Pharmacopeia and is always an advantageous adjunct to this class of remedies. Of course, it must only be taken with the meals and in

no case should more than half a bottle be permitted with the meal. In this quantity, the amount of alcohol is very small.[39]

Although the articles aimed to give a scientific analysis of the therapeutic value of wine, each instalment also provided information on sourcing the best vintages and brands. For example, an analysis of white Bordeaux wines used 'an excellent Sauterne 1870 from The Cafe Royale' to highlight the therapeutic qualities of that particular type of wine.[40] Another article in *The Lancet* in 1894 looked at the medical value of 'tonic' champagnes such as Laurent-Perrier Grand Vin Brut Champagne Sans Sucre and Coca Tonic Champagne Sans Sucre which were recommended for use in treating diabetic patients. Chemical analyses of both drinks concluded that they were palatable and of a similar quality to other 'high class' champagnes.[41] Although there was no medical consensus on the therapeutic value of alcohol as a generic drug there did seem to be some agreement that if alcohol were to be used, it should be of the best quality and type. This is hardly surprising, given that most doctors were middle-class men and many of their fee-paying patients were also middle and upper class. The range of illnesses that were financially treatable with a 'sound claret', coca champagne or a good quality brandy were therefore likely to be middle or upper-class illnesses such as fatigue, neurasthenia, exhaustion from overwork and digestive complaints. In this sense, doctors were only prescribing the types of alcoholic drinks that their patients would normally drink anyway, so in effect it was a prescription to drink *well*.

The financial aspect of prescribing alcohol was perhaps more of a concern for public hospitals and asylums that had to justify expenditure on the poorer working classes. The Glasgow hospital and asylum records show a general decrease in spending on alcohol during a period when it's continued use within medicine courted controversy. Although some doctors wanted to distance the profession from the moral taint of intemperance, many were prepared to carry on prescribing alcohol because they had faith in its therapeutic value. One important point to consider is that alcohol was still being bought and used within hospitals and this suggests a lack of viable alternatives at that time. In other words, doctors simply had no other choice but to prescribe alcohol and perhaps the real pressure was to do so judiciously. This could certainly account for the decrease in the use of alcohol in the decades leading up to the First World War.

NOTES

1. Boothroyde J. S. 'Medicated Wines and Alcohol Addiction': *British Journal of Inebriety*: Volume 7:3: 3 January 1910: p. 146.
2. Ibid.
3. Curth L. H. 2003. 'The Medicinal Value of Wine in Early Modern England': *Social History of Alcohol and Drugs*: Volume 18.
4. 'The Call to Drink': *British Journal of Inebriety*: Volume 5:1: July 1907.
5. Ibid.
6. Barr J. 'Alcohol as a Therapeutic Agent': *British Medical Journal*: 1 July 1905.
7. Ibid.
8. Ibid.
9. Kerr N. 'Ought We to Prescribe Alcohol and How?': *The British Medical Journal*: 5 September 1885.
10. Macfie C. 'On the Duty of the Profession with Regard to Alcohol': *The British Medical Journal*: 22 September 1899.
11. Ibid.
12. 'Alcohol in Workhouses and General Infirmaries': *The British Medical Journal*: 24 May 1890.
13. Macfie C. 'On the Duty of the Profession with Regard to Alcohol': *The British Medical Journal*: 22 September 1899.
14. Ibid.
15. MacDonald J. 'An Address on the Remedial Use of Alcohol': *The British Medical Journal*: 30 July 1909.
16. Ibid.
17. Ibid.
18. Ibid.
19. Ibid.
20. Cage R. A. 1987. 'Health in Glasgow', in (ed.) Cage R. A. *The Working Class in Glasgow 1750–1914*: Kent: Croom Helm: pp. 56–77.
21. NHS Archives (NHS): HB142/8: Glasgow Royal Infirmary Annual Reports: 1871–1914.
22. Thirty-Seventh Annual Report of the Registrar General for Scotland: http://www.histpop.org/ohpr/servlet/PageBrowser?path=Browse/Registrar%20General%20%28by%20date%29&active=yes&m-no=660&tocstate=expandnew&display=sections&display=tables&dis-play=pagetitles&pageseq=38&zoom=5: accessed 1/2/2016.
23. NHS: HB13/51-80: Gartnavel Royal Asylum Annual Reports: 1875–1885.
24. NHS: HB6/3/2: Western Infirmary Annual Reports: 1880–1905.
25. NHS: HB24/3/2: Hawkhead Asylum Annual Reports: 1907–1913.

26. NHS: HB13/5/125: Gartnavel Royal Asylum: Patient Case Notes: James Mackay: January 1888.
27. NHS: HB/3: Gartnavel Royal Asylum Annual Report: 1871.
28. Chrichton Royal Infirmary Archives: CRI 1989.139: Case of Thomas Hoare admitted August 1886, single gentleman, age unknown.
29. NHS: HB65/11: Annual Report of Belvedere Hospital: Medical Superintendent's Report: 1866.
30. Ibid.
31. NHS: HB65/11: Annual Report of Belvedere Hospital: Medical Superintendents Report: 1866.
32. 'Alcohol in Fever': *The British Medical Journal*: Volume 1:8 May 1880: p. 687.
33. Ibid.
34. Ibid.
35. NHS: HB14/2/8: Glasgow Royal Infirmary Annual Reports: 1871–1891.
36. Calculated Using The National Archives Currency Converter: http://www. nationalarchives.gov.uk/currency/results.asp#mid: accessed 12/12/2015.
37. 'The Lancet Commission on the Medical Use of Wines': *The Lancet*: 26 June 1880.
38. Ibid.
39. 'The Lancet Commission on the Medical Use of Wines': *The Lancet*: 24 July 1880.
40. Ibid.
41. 'Analytical Records Form the Lancet Laboratory': *The Lancet*: 13 January 1894.

CHAPTER 10

Drinking for Health:
Proprietary Tonic Wines

To the medically uneducated public [meat and malt wines] undoubtedly seem a most promising combination: extract of meat for food, extract of malt to aid digestion, port wine to make blood - surely the very thing to strengthen all who are weak and to hasten the restoration of convalescents. Unfortunately, what the advertisements say – that this stuff is largely pre-scribed by medical men – is not wholly true.[1]

In an article in *The British Medical Journal* in 1898, Dr F. C. Coley argued that doctors should warn patients and the general population to be wary when buying meat and malt wines. The problem with tonic wines was that they made bold therapeutic claims about the health-giving properties of alcohol based on flimsy medical evidence. Although the therapeutic use of alcohol was generally supported and propagated by doctors who wrote prescriptions for alcohol, it was important that its therapeutic use remains within the boundaries of medical control and not be thrown open to 'the medically uneducated public.' In other words, alcohol still had a place in medicine but the general public could not be trusted to use it wisely or responsibly. Yet despite the reservations of the medical profession, tonic wines were a commercial success and the idea of drinking for health was popular among alcohol consumers.

Foley's argument highlights one of the main concerns about the mar-keting of tonic wines expressed by the 1914 Commission on Patent Medicines, which investigated the supposed endorsement of these

© The Author(s) 2018
T. Hands, *Drinking in Victorian and Edwardian Britain*,
https://doi.org/10.1007/978-3-319-92964-4_10

products by the medical profession. The committee was acting upon eth-
ical and moral concerns about the promotion of alcohol consumption
for medical reasons. Dr Mary Sturge was called as an expert witness with
professional experience on the effects of medicated wines. She was asked
her opinion on why people buy tonic wine

> I think one of the answers is that the advertisements are most extremely
> attractive and alluring. I have brought a group of advertisements here ...
> One advertisement states that 'Wincarnis is a natural nerve and brain food'
> ... I do not consider that anything which contains twenty percent of alco-
> hol, which is a nerve depressant and a nerve irritant, has any claim to be
> called a brain food. Then there is the advertisement: 'Nurse? One moment
> please. Wincarnis gives a strength that is lasting because in each wineglass-
> ful of Wincarnis there is a standardized amount of nutriment.' That is cal-
> culated to make people think that it is really a nutritious mixture and when
> it comes to the analysis, we find that the little amount of meat extract is
> nothing approaching the amount of an ordinary cup of beef tea. My point
> is the misleading influence of the advertisements.[2]

Dr Sturge believed that the general public was duped into buying and
consuming tonic wine because they were either unaware of the alcohol
content or believed that alcohol acted as a medium for the delivery of
medicinal agents in the drink. There was no legal compulsion for manufacturers to disclose the alcohol content or ingredients in tonic wine on
product labelling or advertising and these products fell into the category
of 'secret remedies', which the committee defined as proprietary medicines where the labelling contained very little information on the contents and the product advertising made false or misleading claims. It was
known that companies like Coleman and Hall made huge profits from
the sale of their tonic wines and the issue that the committee had to consider was whether the public would continue to buy these products if
they displayed accurate information on the alcohol content and added
ingredients. The manufacturers claimed that by disclosing this information, their products would face increased competition, which would
in turn harm their businesses. The key question for the committee was
whether product labelling was in the best interests of consumers and
this rested on establishing the reasons why people bought tonic wines
in the first place. Dr Sturge shared the opinion that the general public
viewed these products as medicines rather than alcoholic drinks. She
also believed that some people simply did not care to know the alcohol

content or believed that the alcohol content was minimal. She gave the example of her senior nurse

I asked my out-patient superintending nurse what she thought was in Wincarnis and she said "I think it is a nice mixture with perhaps a little alcohol in it." The word win did not mean wine to her, although she is an intelligent woman.[3]

The example of a senior nurse's ignorance over the product labelling was perhaps intended to point the finger of blame towards the manufacturer's misleading advertising (see Figs. 10.1, 10.2, 10.3, and 10.4).

The committee heard evidence from Mr William Rudderham, who was the general manager of Coleman & Co. Ltd., the manufacturer of Wincarnis. The company spent £50,000 annually on advertising the product and Rudderham admitted that the success of Wincarnis was largely due to the ambitious marketing campaign.[4] Coleman's advertised the product in many of the London newspapers such as *The Times, The Star, The Illustrated London News* and *The Penny Illustrated Paper.* The adverts shown are typical examples of those that appeared in national and regional newspapers in England and Scotland. These adverts were themed around the medical uses of Wincarnis as an alleged treatment or cure for a range of physiological and psychological illnesses such as fatigue, brain exhaustion, worry, nervousness, influenza and pneumonia. All of the adverts shown were reliant upon two main strategies to sell the product: one was the use of testimonials from customers and from doctors and the other was the offer of a free sample for the price of a stamp—also known as the coupon system.

Figure 10.1 is typical of adverts that played on concepts of class and gender roles. In the advert, a man is pictured sitting working at his desk while a woman (presumably his wife) brings him a glass of Wincarnis 'by doctor's orders.' The caption claimed that: 'a man who spends his energies recklessly will quickly overdraw his account at the Bank of Health. A man as he manages himself may die old at thirty or young at eighty; brain fag is the foster parent of disease.' In other words, over-work meant an early demise for professional middle-class men and an early widowhood for their wives, unless it was kept in check by a glass or two of Wincarnis. The medical claims of Wincarnis are more obvious in Fig. 10.2, which shows a nurse holding a tray containing an overly large bottle of the product beneath the caption 'The famous winter

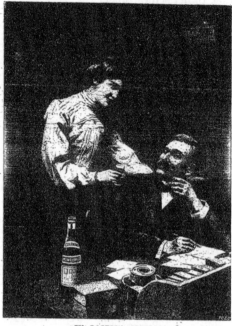

Fig. 10.1   Wincarnis advertisement in *The Penny Illustrated Paper*, London, 1905

wine tonic.' This advert ran in March, perhaps to target people suffering from winter respiratory infections. It claimed that Wincarnis could not only treat winter illnesses but could also be used to prevent them. The

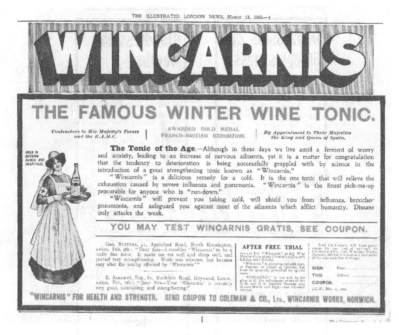

Fig. 10.2   Wincarnis advertisement, *Illustrated London News*, March 1909

medicinal qualities of Wincarnis were further supported by claims that it was used in nursing homes, hospitals and by the Royal Army Medical Corps. This apparent of the product by the medical profession was one of the advertising claims that the committee took issue with. On some Wincarnis labelling it was stated that the product was 'recommended by 10,000 medical men.' When asked by the committee if this claim was based on fact, Rudderham replied that the company had letters from doctors requesting free samples and that these counted as endorsements of the product. In fact, the 'recommendations' of 10,000 medical men were the return coupons for free samples.

Coleman was not the only company using this marketing technique. The committee also heard evidence from Mr Henry James Hall, managing director of Stephen Smith & Co., producers of Hall's Tonic Wine, which differed from Wincarnis in that it contained quantities of coca extract, which was essentially cocaine. Both products were marketed in a similar way, as medicinal wines recommended by the medical profession. Hall stated that: 'Apart from our advertising, the sale of Hall's wine

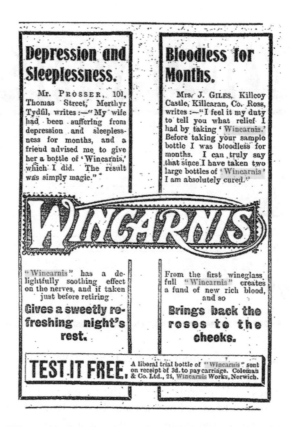

Fig. 10.3   Wincarnis advertisement, *The Penny Illustrated Paper*, London, 1911

is largely influenced by the recommendations of doctors.'[5] To support his statement, he produced letters from doctors and gave these to the committee as proof that doctors who had tried his product had voluntarily given the recommendations. On examining the letters, the committee found that some simply thanked the company for the receipt of free samples. Hall was asked if any of the letters came from doctors who had associations with the company because it was known that a large number of doctors held shares in Stephen Smith & Co. and two doctors were members of the board of directors. Hall dodged this question by reiterating that he had letters from doctors who were not associated with the company. Medical endorsement was the main line of defence used by

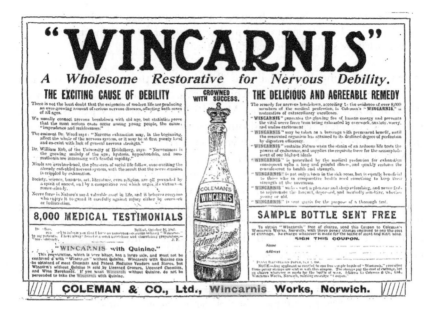

Fig. 10.4   Advertisement for Wincarnis, *The Penny Illustrated Paper*, 1906

both Hall and Rudderham to counter the committee's accusations that they were in fact knowingly selling alcohol under the guise of a medicine and worse still, that their products were recommended for use by women and children. Some of the Wincarnis advertising did specifically target women, mainly for obstetric and gynaecological complaints but also for psychological problems. For example, an advert for 'Coleman's Delicious Wincarnis' that appeared in the *Penny Illustrated Paper* in May 1908 stated: 'For the housewife: When mother's patience is taxed to the uttermost by domestic worries and she is almost ready to faint, Wincarnis is comforting and sustaining.'[6] When asked if he considered it to be morally questionable and physically harmful to encourage women and children to drink alcohol, Hall stated that

> This (his product) is recommended as a tonic and a restorative and when it has effected its purpose, these people do not continue to take it. They are not going to give three shillings and sixpence for a bottle of wine which does not do them any good. I say that in the case of these people who

require the wine, who have been recommended to take the wine by medical men or have been directed to take it by our advertisements, after it does what we state, they leave off taking it.[7]

When questioning both Hall and Rudderham, the committee referred to analyses of their products, which appeared in articles in *The British Medical Journal* in March and May 1909. The articles published the results of chemical tests carried out on some of the most popular brands of proprietary tonic wines, as shown in Fig. 10.5.

Although not pitched as exposés, the articles revealed that most brands of tonic wines contained high levels of alcohol and very little else. Rudderham was asked if he believed that people, and particularly women, bought Wincarnis in the belief that it was a medicine that did not contain any alcohol. Rudderham replied that it clearly stated on the bottle that it was a wine and that 'three small wineglassfuls should be taken daily' and therefore he found it hard to believe that there could

The percentages of alcohol, sugar, and meat extract, and the amount of pure alcohol contained in a wineglassful, may be tabulated as follows:

Wine.	Alcohol by Volume.	Sugar by Weight.	Meat Extract by Weight, corresponding to Nitrogen Found.	Pure Alcohol in a Wineglassful.
				Fl. Drachms.
Claret	9	0.25	—	1½
Hock	10	Trace	—	1½
Champagne(dry)	10 to 15	Trace to 2	—	1½ to 2
Sherry, dry ...	18	0.2 ⎫	—	3 to 3½
„ brown...	23	1.0 ⎭		
Port	20	2 to 6	—	3¼
Bovril	20.15	10.2	0.5	3¼
Lemco	17.26	12.8	0.6	2¾
Wincarnis ...	19.6	18.2	1 2	3
Glendenning's ..	20.8	10.6	0 4	3½
Bendle's ...	20.3	8.0	2.5	3¼
Bivo	19.2	11.5	3.4	3
Vin Regno ...	16.05	7.4	0.3	2½

Fig. 10.5 Chemical analysis of tonic wines: *The British Medical Journal*, March 1909[8]

be any confusion over the alcohol content of the product. However, Dr Sturge provided statements from doctors and temperance groups which suggested that people were buying and consuming tonic wine in the belief that it was non-alcoholic. In one case, a women's temperance group known as The White Ribboners, complained that 'many' of their members had drank tonic wine but were entirely oblivious to the alcohol content. In another case, a doctor from Leeds reported that one of his female patients began drinking Wincarnis when she was 'run down' after her second pregnancy. The woman continued to drink it in increasingly large amounts before moving on to drink spirits instead. At which point she reportedly became 'hopelessly insane.'[9] Dr Sturge argued that women drank medicated wine on a daily basis because they believed that the products provided strength and nourishment during and after pregnancy and childbirth. She essentially implied that women would only drink for health reasons and not for the purposes of pleasure or intoxication. Another witness, Mr John Charles Umney, managing director of the firm that produced Marza Tonic Wine, made the point that the word 'wine' in tonic wine indicated an alcohol content. Moreover, anyone who drank tonic wine would know that it produced a physiological effect. In other words, they would feel slightly drunk.

The issue of intoxication was central to the committee's deliberations on the labelling and advertising of tonic wines. Despite evidence to the contrary, it must have seemed unlikely that men and women who purchased bottles of Hall's Tonic Wine or Wincarnis were completely unaware of any alcohol content. It may have seemed more likely that people did not know of the relatively high alcohol content or the very small amounts of 'medicinal' ingredients contained in the drinks. Depending on the reasons for drinking, intoxication was either the intended primary effect or simply a side effect of the drink. In any case, the commercial success of tonic wine was unlikely to have been based on the belief that it was a non-alcoholic medicine. Most people would have known it was wine and because it was sold as a medicinal drink, people could consume alcohol for health reasons. In the case of women of all social classes, tonic wine provided a socially acceptable way to purchase and consume alcohol in private, for their own purposes and beyond the male gaze. For middle-class men and women, tonic wine perhaps offered an intoxicating relief from the pressures of work or domesticity. In this sense, Wincarnis and other tonic wines created a viable means of intoxication by promoting the idea of drinking for health reasons.

Tonic wine also provided a means of self-medication for people who could not afford to see a doctor or would not see a doctor for trivial ailments. In the last half of the nineteenth century, people were bombarded with adverts for various brands of tonic wines. An Internet search of the British Newspaper Archive for 'tonic wine' generated the highest number of results in the period from 1850 to 1899.[10] Most of these results were for advertisements that appeared in national and regional newspapers across Britain. Alcohol producers, wine and spirit merchants, licensed grocers and chemists were most likely to place adverts. For example, there was an advert in *The Burnley Express* in February 1892 for 'Wilkinson's Orange Quinine Tonic Wine', which was described as 'pure genuine wine of the Seville orange' and was recommended for use in treating influenza, debility and loss of appetite. The wine was sold in all Co-operative stores in Burnley 'at very low prices'.[11] Quinine was a popular additive to tonic wine, not only because of its supposed health-giving qualities but also because of its flavour, which was often described as pleasantly bitter or refreshing. Another advertisement for quinine wine appeared in *The Pall Mall Gazette* in July 1899. The advert was for 'Quinquina Dubonnet' which was described as an 'appetizing, stimulating and strengthening tonic wine of the most delicious flavour made solely from Old Muscat wine and Mexican Quinquina.'[12] Dubonnet Tonic Wine was developed by a French chemist during the French conquest of North Africa in the 1830s. It was designed to encourage the legionnaires to take quinine in a palatable form in order to combat malaria.[13] Another popular ingredient in tonic wine was coca extract, which was sometimes coupled with quinine. An advert for 'Coca and Cinchona (quinine) Wine' appeared in *The Bath Chronicle* in January 1889. The wine was intended for use in treating cases of neuralgia and was available from a local chemist in Bath.[14] Chemists often advertised various brands of tonic wines. One advert that appeared in *The Arbroath Herald* in June 1898 promoted the sale of 'wines for invalids' and listed various brands of meat and malt wines, invalid port and coca wine.[15] Some of the most widely advertised tonic wines were Hall's Tonic Wine and Mariani Wine. The adverts provide examples (Figs. 10.6 and 10.7).

There was profit in selling alcohol as a tonic and companies such as Hall were not the only ones to use this tactic. In the late Victorian period, W & A Gilbey, one of the leading wine and spirit merchants in Britain, stated in its 1897 company report that inserting the word

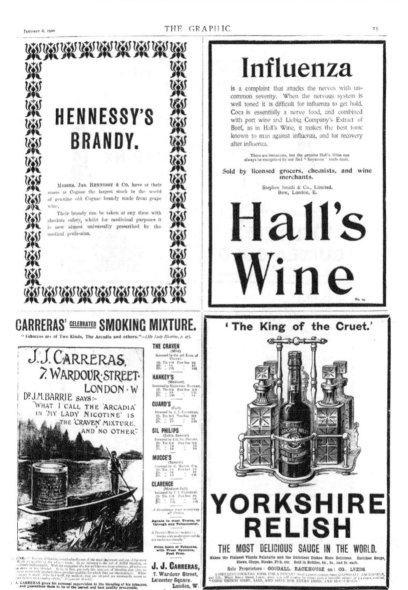

Fig. 10.6   Advert for hall's wine: *The Graphic*: 6 January 1900

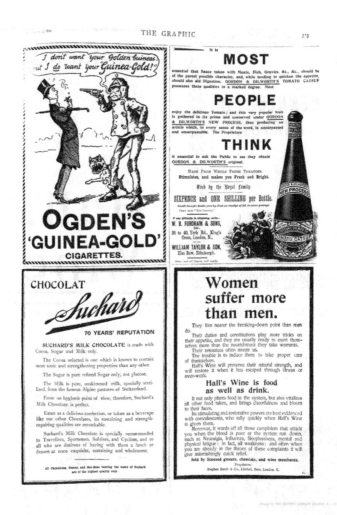

Fig. 10.7   Advert for hall's wine: *The Graphic*: 2 September 1899

'invalid' onto the labelling of various ports, wines and champagnes, had greatly increased sales of these products.[16] Gilbey had used this marketing strategy for a number of years and the 1885 price list included a large section on 'special wines for the use of invalids' which contained invalid champagnes, meat and malt tonic port, quinine sherry, coca wines and invalid port—all sold under the company Castle brand name. One advert for Castle Invalid Port contained an extract from an 1885 article in *The Times* which claimed

> Dr Hood says: "there is no more wholesome wine than genuine port when it is well matured. Two or three glasses daily of such wine will act as a grateful stimulant to the stomach and will assist digestion. Dr. Mortimer Granville states: "stimulants are almost always, I believe, necessary in cases of gout tendency and during the intervals of these attacks. I impose no restrictions except that all alcoholic beverages shall be taken with food and that new or imperfectly fermented wines shall be avoided.[17]

An 1892 sales report stated that in a recent influenza epidemic, more than 200,000 bottles of invalid wines and champagnes had been sold. This gives some sense of the popularity and reliance upon alcoholic substances as medicinal tonics. Doctors still prescribed alcohol as a medicine and consumers also used it as a means of self-medication. It is hardly surprising that the drink trade capitalised on this and marketed products accordingly. As a tonic, alcohol could be drunk moderately and respectably to alleviate a myriad of psychological and physiological problems. This was an attractive idea—particularly for certain groups of consumers who could not otherwise drink without incurring social and moral disapproval. Yet the idea that alcohol was a tonic divided the opinions of the medical profession, and the claim that Wincarnis was endorsed by 'thousands of medical men' was based on very thin evidence. The company could, however, have legitimately claimed that the medical profession still relied upon wine in the treatment of disease and illness. The use of alcohol in medicine not only held commercial value but it also shaped public opinion on the substance and thus partly influenced consumer choices. From a consumers' perspective—if doctors were prescribing alcohol and companies were selling it as a preventative and cure-all for virtually all forms of ill health, then it must have been very tempting to turn to alcohol for comfort and relief. The tonic wine boom is perhaps proof of that.

NOTES

1. Dr F. C. Foley: 'Medicated Wines': *The British Medical Journal*: Volume 2:715: 10 September 1898.
2. House of Commons Parliamentary Papers (HCPP). 1914: 414: Report of the Select Committee on Patent Medicines: Evidence of Dr Mary Sturge.
3. HCPP. 1914: 414: Report of the Select Committee on Patent Medicines: Evidence of Dr Mary Sturge.
4. HCPP. 1914: 414: Report of the Select Committee on Patent Medicines: Evidence of Mr William Rudderham.
5. HCPP. 1914: 414: Report of the Select Committee on Patent Medicines: Evidence of Mr Henry James Hall.
6. 'Coleman's Delicious Wincarnis': *Penny Illustrated Paper*: London: 23 May 1909.
7. HCPP. 1914: 414: Report of the Select Committee on Patent Medicines: Evidence of Mr Henry James Hall.
8. 'The Composition of Some Proprietary Dietetic Preparations': *The British Medical Journal*: Volume 1:795: 27 May 1909.
9. HCPP. 1914: 414: Report of the Select Committee on Patent Medicines: Evidence of Dr Mary Sturge.
10. The British Newspaper Archive: http://www.britishnewspaperarchive.co.uk: accessed 1/3/2016: The search results were: 1800–1849 = 12,661; 1850–1899 = 274, 952; 1900–1949 = 58.
11. The British Newspaper Archive: *The Burnley Express*: 10 February 1892.
12. The British Newspaper Archive: *The Pall Mall Gazette*: 7 July 1899.
13. 'Who Still Drinks Dubonnet?': http://news.bbc.co.uk/1/hi/8159201.stm: accessed 1/3/2016.
14. The British Newspaper Archive: *The Bath Chronicle*: 24 January 1889.
15. The British Newspaper Archive.
16. Diageo Archives: 100433/1: W & A Gilbey Committee Minutes: 1897.
17. Diageo Archives: 100422/190: Gilbey Price List: 1870.

CHAPTER 11

Neither Carnival nor Lent: Everyday Working Class Drinking

The true role of drinking in Edwardian Britain was much more humdrum. Beer was the basis of leisure. It took the place which later became filled with cigarettes and television. Children would fetch jugs from the pubs for tired parents to relax at home at the end of the day. At funerals, at weddings, at harvest, at the initiation of apprentices, at ordinary work breaks, a glass of beer would be exchanged.[1]

For most of the nineteenth and early twentieth centuries, moral and political concerns about alcohol consumption rested on the types of working-class drinking behaviour constantly on show in pubs and on the streets. Yet as the quote above suggests, there was another side to working-class drinking where alcohol formed an ordinary part of everyday life. The quote is from Paul Thompson, a sociologist who conducted an oral history study of Edwardian family life.[2] By stepping into the private world of the family, Thompson's study revealed a culture of 'everyday' drinking among ordinary people. Accounts of excessive drinking were widely documented in the press and in official reports, yet the more humdrum, routine and private drinking habits that existed across the social spectrum largely escaped public scrutiny.

The chapter draws upon an analysis of oral history transcripts which offer glimpses of the ways in which working-class men and women consumed alcohol and their reasons for doing so. This is not a 'top down' vision of working-class drinking skewed by political motives or temperance ideology. Instead, it offers first-hand accounts of drinking

© The Author(s) 2018   129
T. Hands, *Drinking in Victorian and Edwardian Britain*,
https://doi.org/10.1007/978-3-319-92964-4_11

based upon the experiences and memories of surviving Victorians and Edwardians. Many contemporaries (and some historians) looked no further than the publicly drunken aspects of Victorian working-class drinking culture that seemed to be evident on city streets or in pubs, theatres and dance halls. Joseph Gusfield argues that this type of 'carnival and lent' analysis of working-class drinking can be traced to the process of industrialisation and the consequent separation between daily work and leisure.[3] As alcohol consumption was less acceptable in the workplace, it became a marker of leisure time—a symbol of free time spent away from work. The drinking culture of the working classes was viewed as 'carnivalesque' precisely because it ran counter to the sobriety, efficiency and self-control demanded by industrial capitalism. Yet for many working-class families, free time was spent at home, where alcohol formed an integral part of the daily routine that signalled the end of the working day.

Leisure time was one of the many aspects explored in Thompson's study of Edwardian work and family life. The research was conducted in the 1970s when it was still possible to interview surviving Victorians and Edwardians in Britain. The study comprised 444 interviews with men and women all born between 1872 and 1906.[4] Thompson endeavoured to provide a representative sample of the Edwardian population based upon the 1911 census. The interviewees consisted of men and women from all social classes and occupational groups who were living in urban and rural regions of England, Scotland and Wales. The interview schedule consisted of a list of questions that included the roles and work of family members, for example cooking, dining, domestic routines and family values. The interviews were open-ended and some of the questions concerned alcohol consumption. The main questions relating to alcohol were

1. Did your mother or father brew their own beer or make wine? (this question was only directed at working-class interviewees).
2. Did your mother or father go to the pub? (this question was put to all the interviewees).

The interviews lasted between one and six hours and therefore the original transcripts are lengthy (a full extract of data from the original transcripts can be found in the Appendix).[5] The questions on alcohol were mostly asked in a set order but a close reading of the interview transcripts revealed that the interviewees sometimes provided additional anecdotal information about alcohol in other sections of the interviews. Both working-class and middle-class people were interviewed and asked questions that related to alcohol consumption and drinking behaviour. The middle-class interviews will be dealt with in the next chapter which considers the private drinking culture of the higher classes.

The Edwardians study is relevant because it goes beyond the 'carnivalesque' drinking culture of the streets to examine drinking in the context of everyday family life where alcohol formed a part of the daily routine. This offers insights into how working-class people thought about drinking and also into the ways in which alcohol was produced and consumed. There is rich qualitative data on attitudes towards alcohol consumption, which sometimes reflect the social and cultural values of different groups of working-class people. Yet the use of oral history transcripts can have potential pitfalls: These were old men and women recollecting events from their childhoods and they may have forgotten or exaggerated details. However, this was a large representative study that interviewed a wide range of people and it is possible to see patterns in the responses, which suggests some accuracy of detail. But accuracy was not the main reason for using the oral history transcripts. The study provides a unique opportunity to 'listen' to what Victorians and Edwardians had to say about alcohol consumption and to set their discussions and views within the social and cultural context of the time. It was not intended to use The Edwardians study to uncover any 'truths' about alcohol consumption but instead to gain deeper insights into different types of drinking.

Another relevant sociological study is *The Pub and the People*, which was a Mass Observation Study conducted in 'Worktown' in the 1930s.[6] Worktown was in fact Bolton, an industrial town in the north of England which had a population of 180,000 people and 300 pubs. The study was conducted over four years between 1938 and 1942 and involved qualitative interviews, observation and the collection of data and statistics. Although the study offers a snapshot of drinking behaviour in the interwar years, some of the interviewees had been alive in the Victorian and Edwardian periods and therefore they brought with them some ingrained drinking habits and attitudes towards alcohol consumption. The interviewees shared their reasons for drinking particular types of alcohol and these reasons offer insights into the ways in which working-class consumers justified their drinking behaviour.

The Worktown study provides a contrast to The Edwardians study because it focuses on the public drinking culture of the pub whereas The Edwardians drinking is largely situated in the home. When combined, these studies provide insights into working-class drinking within different social, spatial and temporal contexts.

For Victorian and Edwardian working-class families, patterns of drinking largely revolved around family life and home consumption of alcohol was as popular as visiting local pubs. Some of the interviewees recalled the daily trip to the local pub to buy dinner beer

> I remember some of the older boys going round to fetch the supper beer – which was a pint of beer for tuppence, you see they [parents] had a glass each out of that for their supper. But none of us were ever allowed to taste it. But the older boys were allowed to go round with the jug in those days – there wasn't bottled stuff and things you see. And it was considered dreadful for a younger person to be in a pub you see – so that it was only the older ones who were allowed to fetch the supper beer – or perhaps my mother or father would fetch it themselves you know.'[7]

Drinking beer with the evening meal seems to have been a common feature of working-class life for both men and women but it was mainly men who went to the pub regularly in the evenings. One interviewee, a man from Essex, was asked if his mother and father drank beer with their evening meal. He only recalled his mother having a half pint of porter every evening with supper and instead his father would visit the local pub in the evenings. When asked if his mother and father ever went to the pub together, he replied that in his town women did not enter pubs and instead were more likely to consume alcohol at home.[8]

In a study of pubs in York in 1900, Seebohm Rowntree observed the gender differences of customers who frequented different pubs in the town.[9] He noted marked variations in the numbers of men and women who went to different pubs located in working-class districts. In the slums and in poorer working-class areas, women drinkers were a more visible presence within pubs. Yet in more affluent working-class areas, women still visited pubs but many went only to fetch the dinner beer. Rowntree noted that these women were 'all respectably dressed and of cleanly appearance' and that within the pubs under observation 'no cases of extreme drunkenness occurred'.[10] Rowntree drew a distinction in terms of respectability between women who drank in pubs and those who drank at home. In those terms, it was not the act of drinking alcohol that challenged feminine norms but rather the location of alcohol consumption. This mattered less for men's drinking behaviour which was governed by different social rules. Working class fathers' drinking revolved around family life and daily routines. Drinking beer with dinner seems to have been common, as was visiting local pubs in the evenings. Interviewees from urban and rural regions of Britain recalled their fathers' regularly going to local pubs and working men's clubs to socialise and to conduct business

> *Interviewee (JF)*: He'd [father] go out and have a drink because at those times—they used to do a lot of business in the pubs, you see, he'd meet different people in these pubs and they'd say, all right Bill, will you make me a suit you see and he'd meet them in these places … And they'd come into this boozer and just pay him a shilling or two shillings—whatever they could afford [for the suit].
>
> *Interviewer*: Did he stick to the same boozer?
>
> *JF*: Oh no he went to several and then some evenings he went to whist drives and they were held at these public houses you know. And he's probably go there perhaps one night or two nights a week.[11]

The Pubs and the People study focused on the pub as a social institution. The study listed the types of activities that people (mostly men) did in pubs. These included: drinking; smoking; playing cards; dominoes; darts and quoits; singing and listening to the piano; betting and talking about—sport, work, people, drinking, the weather, politics and 'dirt' (scandal). The pub was also a venue for a range of other activities such as weddings and funerals, trades union meetings, secret societies, finding work, crime and prostitution, sex and gambling.[12] The study found that for most people in Bolton, 'drink' meant beer (usually the local beer known as 'mild') and that most drinkers' preferences were motivated by price rather than quality, taste or fashion but again there were gender differences in consumption

> Men are guided by price [of beer] first. Women, who often have men pay for them, go more for taste and the externals. It is more 'respectable' for women to drink bottled beer, mostly bottled stout or Guinness, seldom mild.[13]

In order to find out the reasons why people mainly drank beer, the researchers ran a questionnaire competition that offered financial incentives for consumer participation. The top reasons given for drinking beer were 'social reasons' followed by 'health'. The health reasons were broken down into sub-categories

- General health-giving properties—24%
- Beneficial effects connected to work—17%
- Good effect on appetite—14%
- Laxative effect—10%
- Nourishing—6%
- Tonic—8%
- Valuable properties in malt and hops—6%
- Vitamins—6%
- Diuretic—2%

The researchers believed that many of the health reasons given by respondents were a direct result of brewers' advertising and marketing tactics

> Many people use the phrase 'beer is best'. This is a clue to the large number of references to its health-giving properties; phrases like 'it is body building' – 'picks a man up' – are a direct reflection of brewers' advertising. In the days before mass beer propaganda people drank considerably more than they do now. The history of the last hundred years of drinking in England is a history of decline. These [questionnaire responses] definitely show how advertising phrases intended to keep up consumption have become a part of pub-goers mental attitude to their beer. Beer more than anything else has to overcome guilt feelings. That is why advertising is simple, insistent, fond of superlatives, visual and often showing other people drinking the stuff, radiant with good cheer or good looks.[14]

The researchers concluded that consumers were caught in a trap between temperance and brewers' propaganda, which sought to convince people that drinking was either harmful and sinful or healthy and good. Since the pub was such a central aspect of social life, people either consciously or subconsciously chose to believe the brewers hype. The notion that 'beer is best' had become a deeply ingrained and almost unconscious justification for consuming alcohol. Some of the respondents offered their personal reasons for drinking beer. One man aged 66 gave his reasons for drinking beer

> ... because it is a food, drink and medicine to me. My bowels work regular as clockwork and I think that is the key to health. Also lightening affects me a lot, I get such a thirst from lightening and full of pins and needles, if I drink water from a tap its worse.[15]

Aside from health reasons, the study also considered why men in particular drank beer and found that many of these reasons related to concepts of masculinity and heterosexuality. Some men stated that beer 'put lead in their pencil' or alluded to their drinking habits having a positive effect on their sex lives and even improving their marriages. When asked why he went to the pub and drank beer, one man aged 25, described as a 'shop assistant type' replied 'What else can a chap do in a one-eyed hole like this, he'd go off his chump if there were no ale, pictures and tarts.'[16] This explanation perhaps comes closest to situating beer as an escape or a distraction from the monotony of men's daily lives. The idea that beer consumption somehow boosted masculinity and aided sexual function is not something that could be directly attributed to the effects of brewers' marketing tactics. It could have arisen from the masculine environment of the pub and from the ways in which beer was consumed. Most working-class men drank the local draught beer ('mild' or 'best') in either pints or gills (quarter of a pint) and this distinguished them from women who drank stout, Guinness or bottled beers. It also made 'mild' a 'man's drink' that was therefore imbued with masculine qualities. Add to this the largely male environment of the pub—particularly during weeknight evenings when men would 'escape' the home for a couple of pints—and it is hardly surprising that the consumption of beer became associated with an idealised view of male heterosexuality. Many of the male drinkers in the Worktown study were undoubtedly husbands who 'went home to the wife' at night and therefore it still fell within the scope of 'respectable' drinking if beer consumption was viewed as enhancing rather than diminishing their conjugal roles.

The masculine aspect of beer drinking is also evident in The Edwardians study. Most interviewees stated that their fathers drank moderately—one or two pints at most, and few recalled their fathers being drunk. Some also stated that their father would only visit local pubs at the weekends or in the evenings when finances permitted and instead much of their father's drinking was confined to the home. In a study of late Victorian working-class life, Meacham argues that working-class men were divided between teetotallers who stayed at home in the evenings and beer drinkers that went to the pub for a pint or two in the evening.[17] Meacham also believes that working-class men preferred to spend their leisure time in the company of other men and highlights the importance of working men's clubs, which grew in popularity in the late nineteenth century as places where working men could meet, socialise and drink

> There can be little doubt that a working man of moderation, who spent his leisure hours in a well-managed and generally reputable club, was contributing not only to his personal enjoyment but to his neighbourhood image as a respectable and responsible member of the community.[18]

Although this acknowledges the importance of sociable drinking within working men's clubs and pubs in terms of cultivating and reinforcing ideas about masculinity the analysis misses the significance of domestic drinking where men and women drank together. Some of The Edwardians interviewees recalled their parents drinking at home, particularly in regions where it was considered socially unacceptable for women to drink in pubs

> *Interviewer (I)*: What about your mother, did she like a drink?
> *Interviewee (A)*: No.
> *I*: She never went with him [father] to the pub?
> *A*: Oh, good gracious me, not in those days!
> *I*: Respectable women didn't?
> *A*: No.
> *I*: Do you think that none of your mother's friends ever went, either, the people she knew, they wouldn't have gone along?
> *A*: I think that the people my mother associated with would not have gone to a public house.
> *I*: If they wanted a drink anywhere, how do you think they got one?
> *A*: We wouldn't have gone, but Father might have gone down to what is commonly known as The Rats Hole—it was known as The Rats Hole always has been—and he would have taken a jug down and brought a jug of beer back home.
> *I*: And they'd have a drink together?
> *A*: Yes.[19]

In some regions women were not as constrained by gender norms. One of the interviewees recalled how her mother and other local women met every Monday and had a drink together. The interviewee was born in 1898 and grew up as part of a large working-class family in London

> Well on the Monday – she had a few coppers so her and a lot of women used to go out – mother's day they used to call Monday. And they'd dance down in the ground in the building, you know. They'd enjoy themselves. My mother used to play a mouth organ. And we always knew – Monday, oh my mother'd always have a sweet for me when I came home from school but we always knew when Monday came what to expect. No arguments – people'd be happy, all the neighbours, you know, but my mother didn't mix up with them a lot but it was Monday [and] they seemed to go out and have a drink together. They'd put all their coppers together and they'd have this drink between them and – they never used to get drunk, never had that money. But they'd have perhaps one or two drinks, come back and start dancing. Enjoying themselves.[20]

'Mother's day' was a weekly gathering of local women, which involved a trip to the pub followed by music and dancing in the streets. Few of the other interviewees talked of their mothers drinking publicly in this way. Yet this woman made it clear that in her community, it was customary for the local women to get together once a week and have a drink. Perhaps in some working-class areas of London this type of celebratory drinking was considered normal for women. Yet the majority of interviews described working-class women either drinking at home or to going to the pub in the company of husbands or other male family members

> *Interviewer (I)*: You told me your mum and dad used to go out for a drink?
> *Interviewee (LB)*: Oh yes. Yes. That was their treat—yes.
> *I*: In those days were women allowed to go in pubs?
> *LB*: Oh yes. Yes. Yes. The first place—there was—it's a little place—I don't know whether it's still there—It was called The Money up Hodge Lane and—they used to have a sing-song of a Saturday night.
> *I*: There was no prejudice against women going?
> *LB*: Oh no—none at all. And—they used to have a sing-song of a Saturday night.[21]

In some working-class communities, it was considered socially acceptable for women and children to go to local pubs to obtain alcohol for home consumption. One interviewee born in Dorset in 1904 remembered her grandmother's drinking habits and how she used to regularly visit the local pub to get beer to take home and drink with friends

> Now my grandma – I tell you – when I was – how old was I – about twelve or thirteen I suppose – oh she must have been – must have been going on a long time before that, but I can particularly remember – you know they used to wear the capes, the old ladies, and a little bonnet with a – rose in the – or something in the front, and tied under the chin? Well she used to put her cloak on, take her little jug, go down to what used to be The Prince of Wales. Go down there and get a – half pint of stout. Go home, take her bit of cheese, and she used to go down to a friend's called Mrs Tizzard – Emma we called her. And she used to take her bread and cheese and her half pint of stout down there and have that there with Emma. I can see her now. With her cloak and her little jug, you know.[22]

Stout was a popular drink among women, particularly during pregnancy and after childbirth. This popularity could have stemmed from advertising which promoted the health-giving and nutritious properties of beers and stout (see Figs. 11.1 and 11.2).

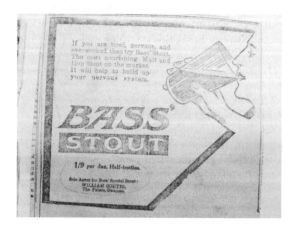

Fig. 11.1 Bass & Co. advertisement c. 1900–1910, Courtesy of The National Brewery Centre[23]

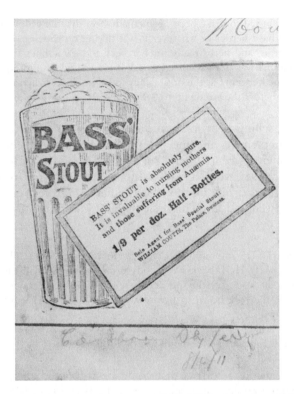

Fig. 11.2   Bass & Co. advertisement c. 1900–1910, Courtesy of The National Brewery Centre[24]

One interviewee who was born in Essex in 1881 recalled his mother drinking stout during pregnancy, even though his father was a teetotaller.[25] Another interviewee who grew up in London had similar memories of her mother drinking small quantities of stout on a regular basis

> I remember mother used to have a bottle – a quart bottle of stout – very reasonable in those days – used to last her a week. She used to have a little drop in a glass like that – and then of course we'd all say to her can we have a little drop.[26]

Bottles of stout and jugs of beer from pubs were not the only ways that working-class women obtained alcohol. It also seemed to be common to brew beer and herbal wines for home consumption. Most of the working-class interviewees were asked if either of their parents brewed or fermented their own homemade beer or wine

She [mother] used to make beer. Homemade beer in a big yellow mug and bottle. And have nettles or whatever it was drying on the line. Drying on the line, nettles and herbs ready for her beer and sometimes she used to tell me before I was born she used to sell it on a Sunday morning to people who came knocking at the door. They loved it. That's when we lived in Manchester before they came up to Salford.[27]

Brewing and selling beer for home consumption may also have been a way to supplement income. Despite regional differences, working-class women from urban and rural areas, made their own beer and wine. In some cases, women made non-alcoholic 'botanic' or herb beer and wine that was drunk by the whole family as a 'tonic' or as a 'treat' but many brewed and fermented alcoholic drinks that were consumed regularly

Interviewer (I): Do you remember your family brewing beer at all?
Interviewee (EP): Herb beer. Everybody brewed herb beer in them days. That was all made of stinging nettles and various seed cones and you had to tie the cork down with wire else it'd blow off. That was always for Sunday dinner.
I: What was it like?
EP: Very good. Wish I had some of it now.[28]

By producing alcoholic drinks that could be consumed at home, working-class women could overcome some of the barriers to drinking posed by gender values. It was perhaps also cheaper to make beer and wine than to buy it from local pubs or licensed grocers. Aside from thrift, there was more privacy in making and consuming alcohol at home and therefore this could have been an attractive option for women who wanted to drink. Yet there was a certain degree of skill involved in making home brew and the cost of equipment and ingredients would have mattered. In A Plain Cookery Book for the Working Classes, published in 1854, there were instructions for making elder wine and homemade beer.[29] Successful fermenting and brewing were dependent upon a fresh supply of clean water, adequate equipment with the space to house it and of course suitable ingredients. Making homemade beer and wine also took time so given these factors and the constraints of money, space and time faced by many working-class families it is surprising that so many of the interviewees recalled their mothers' making alcoholic drinks. As Mitchell notes, for many working-class families, 'dinner beer' was a staple feature of the teatime meal, especially for men coming home from work in the evenings.[30] It may be that the production of homemade alcohol supplemented the beer bought from pubs and if home brew was sold, it added to the household income.

Many of the working-class families seemed to share the same tastes in the types of alcohol consumed and also made similar choices in terms of drinking venues. Beer, ale and stout were all popular drinks. The interviewees were asked about both their parent's drinking habits and it was clear that men and women's access to alcohol and drinking behaviour varied in terms of gender and region. Some stated that one or both of their parents were teetotallers and never drank any alcohol and a few described problem drinking and alcoholism in the family. Yet the majority recalled their parents' drinking habits as being moderate and governed by concepts of respectability and by financial constraints. In some regions it was socially acceptable for women to drink in pubs, in public and in the company of other women but most interviewees described their mothers drinking at home in the company of husbands or other male relatives. The pub was described largely as a masculine space and this was perhaps most evident in the Worktown study where concepts of masculinity governed drinking preferences and behaviour. The majority of interviewees recalled drinking behaviour that revolved around 'normal' and 'everyday' family life. Some spoke of enduring periods of poverty and hardship during their childhoods, yet few attributed their family's economic circumstances to their parents drinking habits. The interviews painted pictures of hard-working fathers and thrifty, capable mothers for whom drinking alcohol was a small but significant part of their daily lives. In these terms, drinking seemed like a banal activity that was guided by the daily routine of family life and governed by financial constraints. There was nothing carnivalesque about this type of drinking; it was not excessive, nor was it pathological. It was simply another humdrum aspect of working-class family life.

NOTES

1. Thompson P. and Lummis T. 1970/2009. *Family Life and Work Experience Before 1918 (1870–1973)*: 7th Edition, Colchester: Essex: UK Data Archive, accessed May 2009: SN: 2000: https://doi.org/10.5255/UKDA-SN-2000-1: pp. 170–171.
2. Ibid.

3. Gusfield J. 1992. 'Benevolent Repression: Popular Culture, Social Structure and the Control of Drinking', in (eds.) Barrows S. and Room R. *Drinking Behaviour and Belief in Modern Society.* California: University of California Press: pp. 76–91.

4. Thompson P. and Lummis T. 1970/2009.

5. See Appendix B for the full list of data extracted from the study.

6. *The Pub and the People: A Worktown Study by Mass Observation.* 1943: London: Victor Gollancz.

7. Thompson P. and Lummis T.: Interview No. 39, female born 1891 in London.

8. Thompson P. and Lummis T.: Interview No. 93, male born 1886 in Essex.

9. Rowntree S. 1908/2016. *Poverty: A Study of Town Life*: London: Macmillan: https://ia800304.us.archive.org/28/items/povertyastudy-to00rowngoog/povertyastudyto00rowngoog.pdf: accessed 16/2/16.

10. Rowntree S.: pp. 325–326.

11. Thompson P. and Lummis T.: Interview No. 321, male born in 1899 from Nottingham.

12. *The Pub and the People: A Worktown Study by Mass Observation* (London: Victor Gollancz, 1943): pp. 10–12.

13. *The Pub and the People*: pp. 10–12.

14. *The Pub and the People*: p. 27.

15. Ibid.: p. 43.

16. *The Pub and the People*: p. 47.

17. Meacham S. 1977. *A Life Apart: The English Working Class 1890–1914*: London: Thames & Hudson Ltd.: p. 29.

18. Ibid.: p. 123.

19. Thompson P. and Lummis T.: Interview No. 23, female from Oxford, born 1905.

20. Thompson P. and Lummis T.: Interview 298, Jane Willsher (born 1898), Housewife from London.

21. Thompson P. and Lummis T.: Interview No. 81.

22. Thompson P. and Lummis T.: Interview No. 382.

23. National Brewing Archive (NBA): Bass Advertising Records: c. 1900–1910.

24. NBA: Bass Records: c. 1900–1910.

25. Thompson P. and Lummis T.: Interview No. 96.

26. Thompson P. and Lummis T.: Interview No. 53, female born 1894 in London.

27. Thompson P. and Lummis T.: Interview No. 47, male, born 1902 from Salford.

28. Thompson P. and Lummis T.: Interview No. 113, male born in London, 1887.
29. Francatelli C. E. 1853/1977. *A Plain Cookery Book for the Working Classes*. London: Routledge: Beer making: pp. 64–67; Wine making: pp. 57–57.
30. Mitchell S. 1991. *Daily Life in Victorian England*: Westport: Greenwood Press: p. 127.

CHAPTER 12

The Drinking Cultures
of the Higher Classes

On the guests being seated at the table: It is not unusual, where taking wine is *en regle* [customary], for a gentleman to ask a lady to take wine until the fish or soup is finished, and then the gentleman honoured by sitting on the right of the hostess, may politely inquire if she will do him the honour of taking wine with him. This will act as a signal for the rest of the company ... at many tables, however, the custom or fashion of drinking wine in this manner is abolished, and the servants fill the glasses of the guests with various wines suited to the course which is in progress.[1]

If working-class drinking can be described as humdrum and routine then in contrast, the drinking culture of the higher classes involved a bit more show and spectacle. There was a desire to consume alcohol in a conspicuous manner in order to reflect and promote social status and the key ways of doing so were to consume the 'right' sorts of drinks in the 'right' kind of places. The quote above from *Mrs Beeton's Book of Household Management* describes the protocol for serving alcohol at dinner parties.[2] For many middle- and upper-class men and women, drinking wine with meals formed an intrinsic part of the daily routine—much like the dinner beer of the working classes. Davidoff argues that imperial notions of civility and social duty governed dining and entertaining, which were the central aspects of Victorian middle- and upper-class social life.[3] The domestic context of alcohol consumption was governed by rules of social etiquette, which both demonstrated and reinforced social class and gender values. Within middle- and upper-class homes purchasing, serving

© The Author(s) 2018   145
T. Hands, *Drinking in Victorian and Edwardian Britain*,
https://doi.org/10.1007/978-3-319-92964-4_12

and consuming good quality wines and spirits were key ways to demonstrate levels of cultural capital and good taste. Writing in 1853, Charles
Dickens observed that

> Nothing in domestic economy tells more of home comfort and conse-
> quently of home happiness, than the quality and condition of the wine
> and the manner in which it is served ... without a good wine, a dinner is
> worthless.[4]

Dickens wrote an article in *Household Words* that offered advice on
purchasing, keeping and consuming wines and spirits. He argued that
despite the glut of domestic cookery manuals, few had tackled the issue
of buying and serving wines to be consumed within the home.[5] Dickens
believed that good quality wines and spirits were a necessary accompa-
niment to dinner and that bad wine was 'abhorrent' to good hospital-
ity.[6] He therefore instructed his readers on how to serve good quality
wines for dining and entertaining. The main wines consumed with dinner were port, sherry, Burgundy, Claret and Hock and when entertaining at evening parties, good quality champagne was served to guests.[7]
Dickens emphasised the importance of sourcing only the best quality
wines and spirits from reputable wine merchants but there were other
retail options.

In the wake of The 1860 Wine and Refreshment Houses Act, the
wine retail market flourished and businesses like the Victoria Wine
Company built a reputation and success through establishing a nation-
wide chain of shops selling good quality wines and spirits.[8] In addition,
the 1860 Act also stimulated the growth of the off-license trade which
lead to the expansion of licensed grocers. Therefore in the second half
of the nineteenth century, good quality wines, beers and spirits could
be purchased in a range of retail outlets. Many middle- and upper-class
homes held accounts with local wine merchants and licensed grocers,
and in most cases, women managed the purchase of alcohol. In *The Book
of Household Management*, Mrs Beeton described wine as an essential
household commodity. Her domestic guide outlined strict rules regarding the use and consumption of alcohol—from wine use in entertaining to paying the servants their beer allowance. For Mrs Beeton and her
middle-class female readership, knowledge of the correct and desirable
use and consumption of wine was essential because domestic dining was
the domain of women and as such it was governed by gendered rules.

For middle- and upper-class women, domestic dining, entertaining and social engagements were some of the few occasions in which it was considered permissible for women to drink alcohol and as with working class women, respectable drinking had to fall under the male gaze—hence the moral panic in the late nineteenth century regarding women's access to alcohol through medical prescriptions and licensed grocers which were both believed to have led to the reported rise in 'secret drinking' among women of the higher classes. Although it was morally permissible for women to drink at some social occasions, there were concerns that they somehow craved alcoholic intoxication more than men and consequently were unable to govern their passions. Following the publication of an article on 'drawing room alcoholism' in *The Saturday Review* in 1871, there was much debate in the press regarding middle- and upper-class women's drinking habits. Many of the regional papers ran opinion pieces speculating on the causes and consequences of the perceived rise in women's drinking

> Women seldom drink for gratification of their palate and the pitiable dram drinker sometimes loathes the spirit she gulps down. Good or bad wine, potato brandy, curacao or gin will satisfy her if only her nervous organisation be sufficiently saturated. The volume of light wine or beer sometimes taken is almost incredible ... The test of safety in the modern use of alcoholic drinks seems to be the power in the persons of fair health to leave off their accustomed beer or sherry without inconvenience or moral effort. This test might be occasionally applied by rational women to themselves or insisted by their mankind.[9]

Dinner parties were some of the few social occasions where middle- and upper-class women could drink for gratification and do so in a manner that was deemed respectable. The same degree of moral scrutiny and control did not apply to the drinking habits of middle- and upper-class men, for whom dinner parties in the home were only one potential site of alcohol consumption. Some of the interviewees in The Edwardians study recalled their fathers drinking and dining in the gentlemen's clubs that were situated in and around Pall Mall and St James's in London

Interviewer (I): Did he [father] belong to any clubs?
Interviewee (LP): Yes.
I: What were they?

> *LP*: He belonged to the Oxford and Cambridge and he belonged to the Carlton and he belonged to the Marlborough. King Edward put him up for The Marlborough and I think he belonged to of course a lot of Conservative Clubs and sort of country clubs and things, those were the London Clubs he belonged to.
> *I*: Did he go to them a lot?
> *LP*: Yes. Oxford and Cambridge he went a lot.
> *I*: On what occasions did he go there? To eat or when they were having a debate?
> *LP*: Oh he went there to eat and very often lunched there and usually went in there in the evening.[10]

For men of the higher classes, gentlemen's clubs offered an alternative to the domestic sphere by providing private spaces for socialising, net-working, dining, drinking and entertaining. In a study of late nineteenth-century London Clubs, Amy Milne-Smith describes gentlemen's clubs as places where middle- and upper-class men forged their class and gender identities.[11] The London Clubs flourished in the nineteenth century and between 1880 and 1914 there were 75 clubs located in the West End of London and all were exclusively for men.[12] Regional gentlemen's clubs also gained popularity in the late Victorian period. For example, The Western Club in Glasgow which was founded in 1825 for the purposes of providing its members with 'cheap and well-cooked dinners' and 'wine free of death in the bottle'.[13] The Western Club was established to cater for the needs of middle- and upper-class men living in Glasgow and the surrounding areas by providing overnight accommodation and a private space for dining and entertaining. Gentlemen's clubs were run as either commercial ventures or more commonly as members-only clubs, which were formed through mutual interests and associations. The most popular clubs with the largest numbers of members were political and military clubs but other clubs were formed through mutual interests in art, literature, sport, travel and school or university affiliation.

Some of the upper-class interviewees in the Edwardians study referred to their fathers as 'club men' meaning that they spent a good deal of their leisure time dining and socialising in one or several of the West End Clubs. Club men were composed of politicians; landed gentry; doctors; businessmen; militarymen; clergymen; and writers and artists. These were men from different social backgrounds who shared a similar desire to socialise privately but also conspicuously within clubs that offered both a means of social escape and a way to cultivate and display social status. Milne-Smith believes that 'clubs were relevant to a much broader spectrum of the population than their members alone and the Club is an entry point into issues of class, gender and social life in Britain.'[14] Gentlemen's clubs are also an entry point into issues surrounding alcohol consumption and the drinking cultures of the upper classes which often escaped public scrutiny.

GUARDIANS OF TASTE: THE DRINKING CULTURE OF VICTORIAN GENTLEMEN'S CLUBS

Most of the private members clubs had organising committees and sub-committees charged with various tasks that contributed to the running of the club. As dining and drinking were central and important aspects of club life, many of the London Clubs had wine committees that were responsible for sourcing, selecting and purchasing the alcoholic drinks sold within Clubs. The archival records of two London Clubs, The Athenaeum and The Reform Club, offer insights into the ways in which the wine committees operated in the late nineteenth century. The Athenaeum was founded in 1824 for the purpose of providing a social venue for gentlemen with shared interests in the arts, literature and science. The Reform Club was established in 1836 and started out initially as a political club for members associated with the Liberal party. By the last quarter of the nineteenth century, both clubs, although founded for different purposes, were attracting men who moved in similar circles.[15] Sir Arthur Conan Doyle was a member of both the Athenaeum and the Reform Clubs and indeed many men held membership of several West End Clubs where they dined and drank regularly.[16] In a history of The Athenaeum Club, written by one of its members Mr F. R. Cowell, the author praised the work of the Club's successive wine committees

> Such a tribute is more necessary because histories of Clubs do not usually have much to say about wine, which matters less because memories of vanished vintages and long-forgotten wine lists can be merely tantalising irrelevancies to those with no hope of profiting from either. That many members of the Athenaeum can recall Cockburn's '27 port and other splendid wines is small consolation to them or anyone else now that stocks are exhausted.[17]

Cowell applauded the 'vigilance and skill' of wine committees in ensuring that 'splendid' and memorable wines were served within The Athenaeum. The club members who served on wine committees were expected to liaise with wine merchants, select and sample various wines, beers and spirits and ensure that the Club was stocked with the best quality alcoholic drinks. In this sense the wine committees acted as guardians of taste within gentlemen's clubs. Bourdieu argues that the consumption of goods is one way in which the concept of taste can be used to define and demonstrate social class status.[18] Bourdieu uses the example of art to show that art appreciation is a decoding operation in which the consumer possesses and uses the ability or education to unlock and understand the meaning or cultural code in a work of art. In a similar way, wine appreciation is also a decoding operation in which the consumer must possess the necessary skills and education in order to make informed judgements on the quality of wine. Educated judgements and appreciation of art or wine require a certain degree of cultural capital that was most evident in people from higher social class backgrounds. Being able to crack the cultural code in objects and consumer goods was a key way to cultivate and display social status and to delineate concepts of good taste.

Bourdieu argues that the taste of the working classes is the taste of necessity and function, whereas the taste of the higher classes is one of liberty or luxury.[19] The wine committees within Victorian gentlemen's clubs were tasked with cultivating and upholding particular standards of taste in alcoholic drinks which mirrored the social status of club members. Although The Athenaeum and The Reform Clubs were formed through mutual interest and associations, the club members were drawn from different social circles and therefore brought with them differing levels of cultural capital which would have either enhanced or diminished their knowledge and appreciation of alcoholic drinks. However, the clubs had certain standards of taste to uphold and adhere to and these tastes did indeed reflect concepts of liberty and luxury. The men who drank in the clubs had the freedom and finances that allowed them to do so and they expected to be served only the finest quality alcoholic drinks. As guardians of taste, the wine committees did indeed exert considerable 'vigilance and skill' in ensuring that the alcohol consumed in The Athenaeum and The Reform Clubs reflected the class and gender status of club members.

The wine committees of both clubs spent a good deal of time and money choosing the 'right' wines, spirits, liqueurs, beers, cigars and cigarettes. Both clubs dealt with several local wine and spirit merchants and purchased various types of drinks from different suppliers. The Reform Club's wine and cigar committee records from 1889 to 1904 contain detailed information on the selection and purchase of alcohol.[20] Committee meetings were held regularly and consisted of dealing with wine merchants, reaching decisions on sample tastings, placing or rejecting orders and managing accounts. The committee sampled different types of wines, spirits, champagnes and liqueurs and orders were based upon the tasting sessions. Effectively this meant that the types of alcoholic drinks sold within the Club were constantly changing. Between 1889 and 1904 The Reform Club dealt with four wine and spirit merchants: Claridge, Cockburn, Alnutt and Campbell. The Club also held accounts with major English brewers such as Ind Coope, Whitbread and Alsopp. The wine list for 1891 detailed the types of alcoholic drinks sold within the Club. The list was organised into categories of drinks, for example: port; sherry and madeira; champagne; claret; Moselle; Burgundy; Chablis and Sauterns; Australian; Hungarian; Italian; Greek; liqueurs; spirits; mineral waters. In each category there were 14 types of port; 14 types of sherry; 37 types of champagne; 10 types of Hock; 35 types of Claret; 5 types of Moselle; 13 types of Burgundy; 2 types of Chablis; 6 types of Sauterne; 6 types of Australian wine; 2 types of Hungarian wine; 5 types of Italian wine and 3 types of Greek wine. The liqueurs and spirits section included: Absinthe; Benedictine; Angostura; Vermouth; brandy liqueurs; Curacoa; brandy; rum; gin; Hollands and whisky—Irish and Scotch. The beers and ales sold were Allsopp; Bass; Burton; Scotch; Whitbreads extra stout; Stout; Guinness; Pilsner Lager Beer; Bass's Ale; Ind Coope's table beer and cider. The wine list also contained information on the vintage, date of purchase and price of the drinks.[21] Another wine list from 1899 contained 2 sections: Club wine and Merchants wine. The Merchants' Wines were marginally more expensive than the Club Wines which were sold to Club members without a significant markup on the retail price—for example, Giesler Extra Super Dry Champagne bought for 6s 7d per bottle was sold in the Club for 7s 9d.[22]

The sale of wines and spirits generated modest profits but greater profits could also be made by investing in stocks of wines that would potentially increase in value and therefore contribute to the assets of the Club. In a history of The Reform Club, Woodbridge states that wine and spirits have always made the largest contributions to the profits from the sale of provisions and claims that the Club's leading assets between 1840 and 1910 were its stocks of wines and spirits.[23] The Athenaeum wine committee operated in a similar way to that of The Reform Club and as Graph 12.1 shows, wise investment in wine generated income for the Club.

The graph shows a fluctuating profit margin from sales of alcohol because periodically, stocks of wine would be put up for sale to Athenaeum Club members. For example in 1900, stocks of 1868 Madeira and 1874 Claret were released for sale and this may have accounted for the larger profits generated from the sale of alcohol in that year. Private clubs were not required to pay excise duties or license fees for the sale of alcohol. In effect this meant that clubs could sell alcohol at any time of day and because there was no payment of excise duties, the alcohol sold within clubs was modestly priced. The absence of excise duties also allowed private clubs to invest in stocks of wine that could then be sold to generate more substantial profits for the club. However, investment in stocks of wine was not without risk. In a contemporary

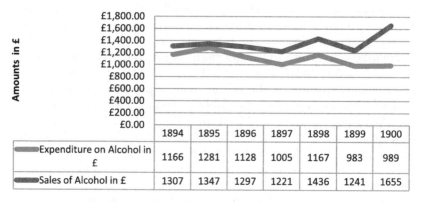

Income & Expenditure on wines, beers & Spirits in The Athenaeum Club

	1894	1895	1896	1897	1898	1899	1900
Expenditure on Alcohol in £	1166	1281	1128	1005	1167	983	989
Sales of Alcohol in £	1307	1347	1297	1221	1436	1241	1655

Graph 12.1 Income and expenditure on wines, beers and spirits in The Athenaeum 1894–1900[24]

account of London Clubs, Major Griffiths outlined the importance of wise investments

> If the [wine] committee elects to depend upon the wine merchants, and buy in small quantities from time to time, it is called upworthy of the traditions of a great club; if the club keeps up a cellar facing the risk of deterioration in a large stock, or a change in taste that makes a particular wine so much dead money, no excuse is accepted for the inevitable loss entailed. One famous establishment not long since disposed of some hundreds of dozens of vintage clarets – high class Clos Vougeot, Lafitte, Mouton Rothschild, and the rest – for a mere song, because they were no longer in demand for after-dinner drinking, on account of the hunger so universally displayed for tobacco. Yet again, when a certain brand of champagne failed for some occult reason to win popularity, it was offered for removal at the price of ginger beer, and the fortunate purchasers obtained a wine which presently so improved by keeping as to rack with the best. No *amende* was made to the sagacious members of the wine sub-committee who had bought it originally.[25]

The wine committees were not only expected to purchase types of alcohol that reflected particular standards of taste but they were also tasked with the risky business of stocking wine cellars that could a generate fairly substantial incomes. Within gentlemen's clubs, the purchase and sale of alcohol were governed by a different set of social and legal rules. The licensing of private clubs was dependent upon the club being either a proprietary or private members club. In proprietary clubs, stocks of alcohol belonged to the club owner who then sold alcohol at a profit to club members—these clubs operated in much the same way as public houses or hotels. Whereas in private members clubs, stocks of alcohol belonged to all the club members who were viewed as being supplied with alcohol rather than being sold alcohol at a profit.[26] This was a legal technicality which allowed private members clubs to escape the licensing laws. It was not until the Licensing Act of 1902 that private clubs were brought under any kind of legal jurisdiction. The legislation required that all private members clubs selling alcohol were registered with local justices but this did not mean that private clubs were regarded as licensed premises and therefore the sale of alcohol within clubs remained unregulated.

Clubland was viewed as a distinctly private sphere where dining, drinking and conviviality could exist without any external interference.

Legal definitions aside, this was also because Clubmen were drawn from the social and intellectual elites. In this sense, the alcohol bought and sold within gentlemen's clubs was viewed as a respectable commodity that was consumed for reasons other than mere intoxication. Arguably, the real value of alcohol was not as an intoxicant or as a social lubricant but as a marker of education and civility. As guardians of taste, the wine committees had their work cut out because the members of The Athenaeum and The Reform Clubs had high expectations of the drinks that they consumed. Major Griffiths believed that Club habitués craved comfort, conviviality and companionship and that they were drawn to gentlemen's clubs because

> The best of everything is at their disposal; material comforts and intellectual delights of the sort that appeal to them. The pleasures of the table are within easy reach; choice fare prepared by a chef who, with a more or less violent stretch of the imagination, is supposed to pass as a cordon bleu; wines of the finest vintages, if they are content to accept the committee's selection, have been laid down for them, offering the widest choice of drinks, and their perpetual absorption, if that way inclined.[27]

The Athenaeum and The Reform Club sold a similar range of alcoholic drinks and indeed both clubs dealt with the same wine merchants: Claridge and Alnutt. However club members did not always appreciate the selection of wines available and it was a common practice within The Athenaeum to write complaints on the reverse side of dinner bills. In 1893, one Club member, Mr Waldegrave Leslie, dined alone at the Athenaeum and drank half a bottle of Pommery Vin Brut and a glass of sherry. However the wine gave him cause for complaint

> I have the honour of being a member of the Athenaeum for a great many years. The wines of the Athenaeum *used* to be obtained from first rate wine merchants. Why are some of these not now employed? I am not a partner in any wine merchants 'firms' – I am not connected with the wine trade in any way whatever. I protest against the liquor called wine supplied by Claridge. Who is Claridge? The so-called Pommery Vin Brut on the other side [of the bill] has never been made in the Champagne region. All Claridge's champagnes are as bad. They are not champagnes.[28]

Mr Waldegrave Leslie was a frequent diner who often wrote scathing remarks on the reverse of his dinner bills regarding the quality of food and drink sold within the Club. The marked dinner bills were kept and passed on to the Executive Committee who dealt with any complaints. The Athenaeum archive holds marked dinner bills from 1888 to 1910 and these provide insights into the type and volume of drinks that upper-class men consumed in the late Victorian period. When dining alone most men drank moderately, perhaps having a glass of sherry, a half bottle of champagne or wine and a glass of brandy and soda. However there were exceptions: one diner in 1891 had a four-course meal washed down with a pint of East India Pale Sherry, a bottle of Perrier Jouet Champagne and a glass of Chateau Leoville wine.[29] Club members of both the Athenaeum and the Reform Clubs sometimes hosted dinner parties where guests or 'strangers' were invited into the Club for the evening. These dinner parties were usually accompanied with fairly lavish amounts of alcohol. In 1901, Arthur Conan Doyle invited eleven guests to dinner in the Athenaeum where they consumed 2 bottles of Pale East India Sherry; 2 bottles of Rudenheimer; 1 bottle of Chateau Palmer; 8 bottles of Moet Chandon; 2 bottles of Port; glasses of brandy and whisky; and cigars and cigarettes.[31] More formal dinners included a printed invitation which contained the dinner menu, including drinks and toasts. The Reform Club with its affiliation to the Liberal Party hosted prominent dinners where members celebrated political victories. At these sorts of events, the type and quality of food and drink consumed was of paramount importance and only the finest selection of champagnes and wines were served. For example on 8 January 1924, the Reform Club hosted a dinner for members who were successful in the 1923 General Election. The drinks menu included bottles of 1815 Olorosa Sherry; Mumm Cordon Rouge Champagne; Cockburn's 1896 Port; brandy and 'fine Champagne 1865'.[30]

Within the London Clubs, the social status of alcohol consumers went without question—club membership was a badge of honour and an endorsement of elite status. Clubland not only escaped the licensing laws because of the social status of its drinkers and drinking venues; the alcohol consumed within the London Clubs also held an elevated status as a respectable commodity that was consumed for reasons other than mere intoxication. The private drinking culture of gentlemen's clubs was dependent upon more than a legal loophole—it was also very much dependent upon a show of respectability. One key way to achieve this was to select and consume alcohol that was imagined to be the preserve of those with the financial means to afford it and the 'right' amount of cultural capital to be able to fully appreciate it. In a similar way, middle- and upper-class dinner parties also provided social opportunities to display wealth and social status. Knowledge of how to select and serve the best types of alcoholic drinks was important and in this way, alcohol served an important function. Although the drinking habits of the middle and upper classes evaded public scrutiny, the privacy and protection afforded by the home and by gentlemen's clubs did not diminish the conspicuous consumption of alcohol but it did largely evade the spectre of the drunkard.

NOTES

1. Beeton I. 1861. *The Book of Household Management*: London: S. O. Beeton: p. 8.
2. Ibid.
3. Davidoff L. 1986. *The Best Circles*: London: Croom Helm Ltd.: p. 39.
4. Dickens C. 1853. *Household Words*, Volume VIII: www.djo.org.uk/household-words/volume-viii-p: accessed 15/09/2014.
5. Ibid.
6. Ibid.
7. Ibid.: p. 405.
8. Briggs A. 1965. *Wine for Sale: Victorian Wine and the Liquor Trade, 1860–1984*: Chicago: University of Chicago Press: pp. 18–19.
9. 'Drawing Room Alcoholism': *The Ashton Weekly Reporter*: Manchester: 28 January 1871.
10. Thompson P. and Lummis T. *Family Life and Work Experience Before 1918*: Interview No. 2012, Male born 1882 in London. The interviewee was Lord Parmor.
11. Milne-Smith A. 2011. *London Clubland: A Cultural History of Gender and Class in Late Victorian Britain*: London: Palgrave Macmillan: p. 2.
12. Ibid.: p. 28.
13. The Western Club Archives: Wilkinson F. A. *The Story of the Western Club: From Its Inception in 1825 to the Year 1900*: booklet written by a Club member: no date.
14. Ibid.
15. Milne-Smith A.: pp. 12–15.
16. Cowell F. R. 1974. *The Athenaeum: Club and Social Life in London 1824–1974*: London: Heinemann Education Books Ltd.: p. 55.
17. Cowell F. R.: p. 100.
18. Bourdieu P. 1984. *Distinction: A Social Critique of the Judgement of Taste*: London: Routledge: p. xxv.

19. Bourdieu P.: p. xxix.
20. Reform Club Archives (RCA): Wine and Cigar Committee Minutes: 1889–1904.
21. RCA: Wine and Cigar Committee Minutes: Wine List: 1891.
22. RCA: Wine and Cigar Committee Minutes: List of Wines Requiring Selling Price: 1895.
23. Woodbridge G. 1978. *The Reform Club, 1836–1974: A History of the Club's Records*. published by The Reform Club: p. 73.
24. The Athenaeum Archives (AA): Executive Committee Minutes: 1899–1901.
25. Griffiths A. G. F. 1907. *Clubs and Clubmen*: London, Hutchinson & Co.: p. 197.
26. Manchester C. 2008. *Alcohol and Entertainment Licensing Laws*: London: Routledge-Cavendish: p. 334.
27. Griffiths A. G. F.: p. 203.
28. AA: Cat 1/10: Marked Bills: 1891–1897: Complaint of Mr Waldergrave Leslie.
29. AA: Cat 1/10: Marked Bills: 1891–1897.
30. AA: Cat 1/12: Marked Bills: 1901–1903.
31. RCA: Dinner Invitation: 1924.

CHAPTER 13

Conclusions

Drunkenness was only one of many outcomes or reasons that Victorian and Edwardian consumers had for drinking. The desire for intoxication, the multitude of ways to seek intoxication and the range of intoxicated behaviour was infinitely more complex because it was deeply entangled within the social and cultural context in which alcohol was produced and consumed. When Brian Harrison wrote *Drink and the Victorians* he was not particularly concerned with the motives of alcohol consumers and many subsequent historical studies followed suit. The Victorians were however concerned with the motives of alcohol consumers. Questions about alcohol consumption drove parliamentary enquiries, shaped the commercial practices of alcohol producers and sparked debates within the medical profession. The Victorians knew that the problems of alcohol co-existed with the pleasures of drinking and that if alcohol remained a legal intoxicant then the freedom to drink ultimately rested with consumers. While consumer agency existed, people's reasons for drinking alcohol varied and were influenced by broader political, commercial, medical and cultural factors.

The 'great army' of drinkers signalled the beginnings of a consumer society and a mass market for alcohol. Industrial scale brewing and distilling coupled with the rapid expansion of the alcohol retail trade generated more choice for consumers but also fuelled political concerns about widespread drunkenness in towns and cities across Britain. If large sections of the population consumed large volumes of alcohol then it must have seemed logical to expect large amounts of drunkenness. Yet the

© The Author(s) 2018
T. Hands, *Drinking in Victorian and Edwardian Britain*,
https://doi.org/10.1007/978-3-319-92964-4_13

evidence given at the parliamentary commissions on alcohol suggested that people found it difficult to pin down one universal definition of drunkenness since ideas about drunkenness varied regionally and were largely dependent upon the 'three Ds'—the drinker, the type of drink consumed and the drinking location. Alcohol was certainly a route to intoxication but the witness testimonies at the parliamentary enquiries suggest that drunkenness was not the only outcome. This was most evident in the accounts of working-class men's drinking behaviour linked to occupations in the heavy industries and manufacturing. These men were thought to work hard and drink hard and this type of drinking was largely accepted. The public drinking habits of the urban working classes were subjected to moral scrutiny and witnesses gave evidence of large numbers of drinkers frequenting pubs. Working-class Victorians had a vibrant drinking culture with a wide choice of venues and types of drinks. Implicit in the evidence given by police officials was the idea that some public drinking was harmless and that a degree of pragmatism was needed in policing drunkenness. Although less attention was given to the private drinking habits of the working-class men it was largely accepted that some alcohol consumption was normal, for example drinking dinner beer with the evening meal. The Edwardians study offered greater insights into working-class men's drinking that revolved around family life and daily routines. Working-class fathers sometimes visited the pub in the evenings or stayed at home and drank with their wives. The Worktown study focused on working-class pubs and explored some of the reasons men had for consuming alcohol. It showed that drinking behaviour was to some extent shaped by ideas about working-class masculinity.

The parliamentary enquiries were much less concerned with the drinking habits of middle and upper-class men and often the only insights came from the committee members who were alcohol consumers. The heated exchange between the Bishop of Peterborough and Reverend Burns of the UK Alliance during the 1877 enquiry, cut to the core of the debate about the extent of alcohol controls. The very idea of alcohol prohibition was an assault on masculinity because it infringed upon the rights of men (all men and not just working-class men) to consume alcohol. Controlling and restricting the sale of alcohol was one thing but stopping men from drinking in the privacy of their own homes or clubs was, to men like the Bishop, simply absurd. When examining the records of the London Clubs it was clear that alcohol consumption was imagined in a very different way where the status of alcohol was elevated to that of a valued cultural commodity. Bourdieu's ideas about the links between consumption and social class were most evident within the London Clubs where purchasing and consuming particular types of alcoholic drinks demonstrated levels of cultural capital.[1] Victorian men of all social classes were free to drink alcohol because ideas about male drinking and drunkenness were framed by larger debates about liberty versus state control and in a highly patriarchal society the biological and moral freedom to drink alcohol resided with men.

Yet men were not the only alcohol consumers. Women of all social classes drank alcohol. The political enquiries dwelt upon women's drinking—whether it was working-class women drinking out in public or middle and upper-class women drinking 'secretly' in private, it did not seem matter because all women's drinking was deemed problematic. Some witnesses and committee members simply believed that women were worse drunks than men. Yet the interviewees in The Edwardians study gave a different account of women's drinking that was viewed as a part of everyday life. Working-class women made and sometimes sold their own home-brewed alcohol. They drank to socialise or celebrate or sometimes for health during pregnancy and after childbirth. In some regions women drank in pubs or drank at home with their husbands. Middle and upper-class women also drank alcohol as part of everyday life. Dining and entertaining were occasions when it was socially acceptable for higher-class women to consume alcohol for pleasure. The issue of the male gaze—or male power and control exerted over women, may have influenced attitudes towards drinking but it did not curtail women's alcohol consumption. The political and medical concern about grocer's licences demonstrates that some women seized upon the opportunity to buy and consume alcohol for their own private purposes. Working-class women employed in factories and poorer working-class women etching out a living on the margins of society drank alcohol publicly and blatantly. If viewed within the context of women's oppression or conversely women's emancipation, alcohol consumption fits within de Certeau's ideas about a consumer grid of resistance.[2] In this sense, alcohol presented a way for some women to challenge or escape male authority.

The Victorians and Edwardians drank for pleasure but they also drank for pain. The use of alcohol as a treatment in medical practice continued throughout the nineteenth and early twentieth centuries. It was prescribed for a range of physiological and psychological illnesses and

Victorians admitted to hospitals sometimes received treatment with certain types of alcoholic drinks. Debates existed within the medical profession about the efficacy and ethics of prescribing alcohol and there were concerns about therapeutic nihilism—that alcohol did more harm than good, not only to patients but also to professional reputation. Yet it remained an orthodox medical treatment and people held faith in alcohol as a medicine. Some interviewees in The Edwardians study described their mothers drinking stout during pregnancy or after childbirth because they believed it was nourishing and acted as a tonic. The idea of self-medicating with alcohol may have alarmed the medical profession but it was popular among alcohol consumers and this meant that the health benefits of alcohol held enormous commercial value to the drink trade. Marketing alcohol as a tonic was one way to reach consumers and boost sales during a period when the drink trade faced moral and political hostility. By simply rebranding products to include the word 'tonic' on labels, alcohol producers boosted the market and ensured increased sales. The boom in tonic wine sales at the end of the century could not have happened without a receptive consumer market. People had faith in alcohol as a therapeutic drug so all that companies had to do was market products that could treat and prevent a wide range of illnesses. Drinking alcohol for health was not the same as drinking it for pleasure or for intoxication. Consumers could, therefore, drink alcohol 'for health' in a socially acceptable way and the drink trade could sell an intoxicant under the guise of a tonic.

Selling alcohol was a tricky business in the late nineteenth century and in order to be successful, companies had to beat the competition, reach a wide market of consumers and sell them something other than an intoxicating substance overshadowed by the spectre of the drunkard. Fortunately for alcohol producers, the capitalist system supported such practices. Baudrillard's analysis of the manufacturing of needs and desires through advertising and marketing is useful when considering the position of alcohol in the late nineteenth century.[3] If alcohol was only understood in terms of its basic function then it was a potentially dangerous intoxicant that could cause drunkenness and social ruin. If however, it came to symbolise something else, something desirable, then its basic function changed. The challenge for alcohol producers and retailers was to reinvent the substance as something other than a mere intoxicant and James Buchanan did this very successfully with Scotch whisky, which became a drink of the elites. By ensuring that those in positions of power and prestige conspicuously consumed his products, it was possible to turn a common alcoholic drink into a highly desirable cultural commodity. Other alcohol producers such as Bass and Walker also used marketing strategies that created desires and gave consumers reasons to drink their products other than for the purposes of intoxication.

For many people in Victorian and Edwardian Britain, consuming alcohol meant more than simply mainlining intoxication. Alcohol was both an ordinary and an extraordinary substance that constituted an integral part of everyday life. As dinner beer it was the antidote to the toils of the working day. As Scotch, fine wine or champagne it was a marker of social class status. In the hands of the medical profession or indeed commercial interests it was a panacea. In the mouths of women it was a subversive substance. People had many different reasons for drinking other than the desire for intoxicated oblivion. Yet sometimes this was precisely the reason for consuming alcohol. Drunkenness prevailed throughout the Victorian and Edwardian periods just as it does today. The real problem with alcohol is the one alluring quality of the substance—it gets people drunk. Alcohol can therefore be viewed in the same way that Klein considers cigarettes—as a dark, dangerous and sublime intoxicant.[4] The desire for intoxication drives alcohol production and consumption and motivates alcohol consumers to drink in many different ways and for many different reasons.

NOTES

1. Bourdieu P. 1984/2010. *Distinction: A Social Critique of the Judgment of Taste*: London: Routledge.
2. de Certeau M. 1984. *The Practice of Everyday Life*: Berkeley: University of California Press.
3. Baudrillard J. 2003. 'The Ideological Genesis of Needs', in (eds.) Clarke D. B., Doel M., and Housiaux K. *The Consumption Reader*. London: Routledge: pp. 255–259.
4. Klein R. 1993. *Cigarettes Are Sublime*: London: Duke University Press.

APPENDIX

© The Editor(s) (if applicable) and The Author(s) 2018   165
T. Hands, *Drinking in Victorian and Edwardian Britain*,
https://doi.org/10.1007/978-3-319-92964-4

No.	D.O.B.	Gender	Location	Q. 1 Home brewing (HB)?	Q. 2 Parents drinking habits
1	1902	M	Essex	Brewed wine on special occasions	Mother did not drink. Father went to pub occasionally
2	1896	M	Horton	Brewed beer and cider	No pub but drank beer and cider at home
3	1892	F	London	Brewed beer and wine	Father W/M club drank whisky
4	1897	M	London	No home brew (HB)	No pubs/social drinking
5	1888	M	London	Not asked	Not asked
6	1900	F	London	No HB	Parents drank wine at home and went to pub occasionally
7	1887	F	London	Not asked	Not asked
8	1882	M	London	Not asked	Not asked
9	1897	M	Essex	Not asked	Not asked
10	1885	M	Essex	No HB	Bought beer from local farmer who had a shilling license. Men drank beer morning, lunch, dinner. Boys given 'mild beer' with dinner
11	1905	M	Wiltshire	Teetotal	Not asked
12	?	M	Cambridge	Not asked	Not asked
13	1907	F	London	Teetotal	Not asked about pubs
14	1889	M	Essex	No HB but father always had cask of 'four and a half beer' bought from local brewer	Not asked about pubs
15	1886	F	Essex	Not asked	Not asked

(continued)

No.	D.O.B.	Gender	Location	Q. 1 Home brewing (HB)?	Q. 2 Parents drinking habits
16	1882	M	Essex	Brewed own beer	
17	1884	F	Essex	Not asked	Not asked
18	1882	M	Wiltshire	Not asked	Not asked
19	1890	F	Essex	Not asked	Not asked
20	1897	M	Essex	Brewed beer and made wine	Brewed beer at harvest time—'harvest beer'. Farmer paid men and boys in beer also father bought malt and hops with wages to make beer
21	1891	F	Essex	No HB	Well off w/c family. Drank whisky at Xmas and beer with meals. Not asked about pubs
22	1904	M	Essex	No alcohol in house	Father went to pub occasionally
23	1905	F	Oxford	Mother made elderberry wine (alcoholic) drink regularly by parents	I (interviewer): What about your mother, did she like a drink? A: No I: She never went with him to the pub? A: Oh, good gracious me, not in those days! I: Respectable women didn't? A: No
24	1882	M	Staffs	Not asked	Father a 'drunkard'. Spent wages on drink. Sometimes went to pub instead of work
25	1896	M	Staffs	No HB	Was in Band of Hope as child and signed the pledge
26	1889	M	Northmub	Not asked	
27	1895	M	Newcastle	Not asked	
28	1897	F	Staffs	Not asked	Not asked about family drinking habits. Was in Band of Hope as child and signed the pledge
29	1891	F	Llandaff	Not asked	Was in Band of Hope as child and signed the pledge
30	1900	F	Staffs	Not asked	
31	1893	M	Staffs	Not asked	

(continued)

(continued)

No.	D.O.B.	Gender	Location	Q. 1 Home brewing (HB)?	Q. 2 Parents drinking habits
32	1898	M	Liverpool	No HB	Parents did not go to pubs
33	1984	M	Bolton	Mother made ginger wine—sometimes alcoholic	Father 'not a drinker'—only went to pub to do business
34	1897	M	Oxford	Not asked	Father went to pub occasionally
35	1900	M	Oxford	Father ran a pub—family lived above it. Mother made lots of different alcoholic wines	Not asked
36	1896	F	Bolton	Mother made beetroot wine	Father went to pub regularly
37	1901	F	Oxford	Not asked	Father went to pub after work
38	1895	F	Oxford	Mother made wine	Had dinner parties—in a humble rural way. Mother served her wine: 'He would serve that. Sometimes she would have, for very special occasions; he might get a bottle of claret just for the dinner. But he, himself, he couldn't normally afford to drink not every day. But all country people, you know, made wines and sort of beer and those sort of things'

(continued)

No.	D.O.B.	Gender	Location	Q. 1 Home brewing (HB)?	Q. 2 Parents drinking habits
39	1891	F	Oxford	Not asked	Father drank regularly: 'No, no, he - he didn't go - perhaps about once a week you know. No, because, I remember some of the older boys going round to fetch the supper beer - which was a pint of beer for tuppence you see and they had a glass each out of that for their supper. But none of us were ever allowed to taste it. But the older boys they were allowed to go round with the jug in those days - there wasn't bottled stuff and things you see. And it was considered dreadful for a - a younger person to be in a pub you see - so that it was only the older ones who were allowed to fetch the supper beer - or perhaps my mother or father would fetch it themselves you know, remember a lot about that'
40	1892	F	Wooton	Teetotal family	
41	1890	M	Durham	Not asked	
42	1893	M	Oxford	Not asked	
43	1901	M	Liverpool	No HB	Father went to pub regularly. Mother teetotal
44	1888	F	Liverpool	No HB	Father did not go to pubs
45	1896	F	Salford	No HB	Not asked
46	1898	F	Liverpool	Mother made wine—her 'home brew'	Not asked
47	1902	M	Salford	Mother used to make beer	Father went to pub occasionally
48	1894	M	Surrey	Father brewed beer sometimes	Father went to pub regularly. Mother never drank
49	1890	M	Liverpool	Parents ran a pub. They lived above it	
50	1891	F	Surrey	Teetotal family	

(continued)

(continued)

No.	D.O.B.	Gender	Location	Q. 1 Home brewing (HB)?	Q. 2 Parents drinking habits
51	1891	F	Liverpool	No HB	Father did not go to pub. Was in Band of Hope as a child
52	1897	M	Salford	No HB	I: Did they brew beer for the family? JL: No he used to go out for it—used to go out. From the top of Ordsell Lane to where I lived there must have been a dozen pubs. One at every street corner—I can't think of all the names now but—one that me father used to go in was The Liars Arms and it was the corner of where we lived and it's so strange that today—I collect a bit of coal money at week end for a gentleman who has opened—got a public house down there called The Albion—and mother used to go in there at night with about ninepence for a gill and come out drunk 'cos everybody treated her
53	1894	F	London	No HB but mother used to have a quart bottle of that lasted her a week	Father went to pub occasionally. Mother went to music hall occasionally
54	1895	M	Bolton	Mother made herb beer	Father a 'temperance man' active in trades unions but had to go to pubs for meetings
55	1892	M	Salford	No HB	Mother had friend that ran a pub so she went there regularly. Father never went to pub but drank beer at home. Children had to fetch his beer from pub
56	1889	F	Surrey	Not asked	Parents never went to pub
57	1891	F	Surrey	Not asked	Parents never went to pub
58	1889	M	London	Not asked	Father went to pub regularly—'tuppence a pint'
59	1878	F	Essex	No HB	Not asked
60	1892	M	Surrey	No HB	Father went to pub regularly. Mother went to pub after she did the weekly shopping
61	1873	F	Salford	No HB	Father went to pub on a Saturday

(continued)

No.	D.O.B.	Gender	Location	Q. 1 Home brewing (HB)?	Q. 2 Parents drinking habits
62	1901	M	Wales	No HB	Father went to pub sometimes for 'a half'
63	1890	M	Surrey	No HB	No pubs
64	1903	F	London	Mother made ginger wine	Did not mention pubs. Was in Band of Hope as a child
65	1879	F	London	Mother made grape wine	Father went to pub occasionally
66	1887	F	Surrey	No HB	No pubs—parents 'couldn't afford it'
67	1901	M	Bolton	No HB	Father went to pub
68	1883	F	Salford	No HB	Father never went to pub 'he always had his drink at home'
69	1886	F	Swinton	Mother made crab apple wine and brewed herb beer—bought packets of herbs	Not asked
70	1899	M	Essex	Not asked	No pubs mentioned
71	1896	M	London	No HB	Father teetotaler
72	1891	F	Bolton	Not asked	
73	1877	F	Lancs	Mother made redcurrant wine and herb beer	Father went to pub occasionally. Mother went to pub in later life
74	1898	M	Liverpool	No HB	Father went to pub regularly—'liked his pints'
75	1901	F	Manchester	No HB	
76	1895	F	London	No HB	No pubs
77	1896	M	Liverpool	No HB	Father liked a drink and went to pub
78	1887	F	Bolton	Not asked	Father and mother drank in pub
79	1904	F	Liverpool	No HB	Not asked

(continued)

(continued)

No.	D.O.B.	Gender	Location	Q. 1 Home brewing (HB)?	Q. 2 Parents drinking habits
80	1894	F	Liverpool	No HB	Not asked
81	1897	F	Lancs	Father brewed beer	I: You told me your mum and dad used to go out for a drink? LB: Oh yes. Yes. That was their treat—yes I: How many evenings a week did your father spend at home? LB: Well it—he always—was at home. It was just weekend that they went out. Oh yes, because—they were very methodical—very methodical I: In those days were women allowed in pubs? LB: Oh yes. Yes
82	1889	M	Guildford	No HB	Father went to working men's club on a Saturday and also went regularly to the pub
83	1900	M	Guildford	No HB	Not asked
84	1887	M	London	No HB	Not asked
85	1883	F	Essex	No HB	Parents did not go to pub
86	1900	M	Liverpool	No HB	Parents were 'temperate'—went to Band of Hope as a child
87	1889	F	Bolton	Not asked	Father was a 'lifelong teetotaler' and was in a temperance band
88	1885	M	Liverpool	No HB	Father did not drink. However step father did drink and this lead to mother 'enjoying herself' more and having a drink
89	1904	M	Salford	No HB	Not asked
90	1885	M	Salford	No HB	Father always went to the beer house. Mother never drank. First job was in coal mines—was paid in the pub: I: This was a pub? AT: That's the Britannia. The pub—it was called the Britannia. That I: You got paid there? AT: Got paid inside there—with the corty master—used to—at the Friday he used to get all the money from the pits for the coal what we'd turned out and he used to pay 'em out you see

(continued)

No.	D.O.B.	Gender	Location	Q. 1 Home brewing (HB)?	Q. 2 Parents drinking habits
91	1894	M	Guildford	Mother made wine	Was in temperance club as a child: *I:* Did the Church run any temperance club? *TW:* I think it did, but we didn't belong to one. I think they had what was called the Band of Hope, which was a temperance body, but while we were lectured in sermons on temperance I don't recall participating in anything. But we were not … Drink was not discouraged, although my mother made wine at home Father did not go to pubs
92	1897	F	Essex	No HB	Mother had an 'ordinary glass of beer'. Father went out in the evening bit did not specify pub

(continued)

(continued)

No.	D.O.B.	Gender	Location	Q. 1 Home brewing (HB)?	Q. 2 Parents drinking habits
93	1886	M	Essex	*I:* Did she or your father brew beer at all? *GR:* Yes, home brewed beer they used to have. Home brewed beer	*I:* Did you drink beer or did your father and mother ever drink beer with the meals? *GR:* I never remember having—them having beer or drink with their—beer with their meals. No. Only mother used to have her half pint of porter every—night for supper. Yes. Half pint of porter *I:* That wasn't brewed by them? *GR:* Oh no, no. That used to come from the public house next door *I:* Who would fetch it? *GR:* Anyone of us. She used to go herself sometimes—only just out and next—next door *I:* Did she ever go and sit there and have it? *GR:* I never knew mother to go in a—except this—sit in a pub—in a public— *I:* Did women sit in pubs in Thorpe? *GR:* Very seldom. Very few *I:* It wasn't considered the right thing? *GR:* No, no. Not there, no *I:* What about your father, did he go to the pub? *GR:* Oh yes. Every night father went to the—every night he went his pub *I:* Was that before he came home? *GR:* Oh no, after he'd had his supper and done his work and done his gardening and all—summertime. He'd go about say nine o'clock or half past and just go down there for his pint or two whatever he had and come— *I:* Did he always go to the same one? *GR:* Same public house, yes
94	1884	M	Essex	Not asked	Not asked
95	1889	F	Liverpool	No HB	Not asked

(continued)

No.	D.O.B.	Gender	Location	Q. 1 Home brewing (HB)?	Q. 2 Parents drinking habits
96	1881	M	Essex	No HB	*I*: Were they both teetotallers or just your father? *WB*: Oh well, father was but—of course, mother wasn't and all the same very, very little you know for instance if—she was going to have a baby she might have a little drop of stout occasionally you know, but I mean not—generally speaking she didn't. See half a glass—if anybody came in—she'd—half a glass of beer with 'em. And talking about beer. If you wanted any beer you—you took a jug to the pub. See? Bottling—well you see here on the pubs now, bottle and jug department. You—you've seen that probably you see. But—people never take a jug now do they? I've never seen anyone—for years *I*: Did she ever go and have a drink in the pub? *WB*: Well—the only time—it'd be—they used to go, two or three of them, they used to be mother and grandfather and—that little old fellow I showed who was a slater. A dear old chap. And—perhaps a sister and brother-in-law you know, they used to—they used to go in the Corner Pin in Strutton ground and—they'd have a drink you know, perhaps on a Saturday afternoon, done their shopping, but, you—know, just before they parted but you couldn't say they—they had much to drink *I*: Would you mother ever go in on her own? *WB*: Oh Lord, no *I*: Wouldn't be considered respectable in those days? *WB*: No. And even if it was she wouldn't go in. Any more than—well, you know. I'm not a teetotaller altogether but I'd go out—I could go out and step out all day without going into a pub. See? But if I met you or some-body I know—oh well, let's go and have a drink *I*: Companionable? *WB*: Exactly

(continued)

(continued)

No.	D.O.B.	Gender	Location	Q. 1 Home brewing (HB)?	Q. 2 Parents drinking habits
97	1898	F	Liverpool	Not asked	Not asked
98	1895	M	Liverpool	Not asked	Not asked
99	1902	M	Liverpool	No HB	Mother was a 'strict rabid teetotaler' so no alcohol in the house and father did not go to the pub
100	1904	F	Manchester	No HB	Not asked
101	1898	F	Liverpool	Not asked	Not asked
102	1898	M	Lancs	Not asked	Father went to pub
103	1882	M	Lancs	No HB	Father went to pub when he could afford it

(continued)

No.	D.O.B.	Gender	Location	Q. 1 Home brewing (HB)?	Q. 2 Parents drinking habits
104	1890	M	Lancs	No HB	Father went to pub: I: Did he ever take you out on your own? RP: Aye, once took me at Wigan. On—they used to have bird singing, lark singing in cages. In Wigan. In a pub—in Wigan. And I went—I went with him. And—used to put a cage—a bird cage down, they used to give it so long to sing then they used to time it, how long it sung. That would go away, somebody else would come with one and put it down. They used—give it so long to sing, time it, put the time down, that away. And that's way how they used to do and them as has done the most time were the winner. I know me dad won a copper kettle with it I: Who provided the prize? RP: This—these public houses—publicity—publicity to get custom you see I: Do you remember what it was like in the pubs as a child? RP: Oh they were all shankies—they were all shankies. No—no— I: What are old shankies RP: Low—low roofs with—with big wooden—wooden whatsits across I: Do you remember any of the people who used to go in the pubs—what they were like and what went on? RP: I only know when me dad went—went in the—when there were bother on—and—landlord sends across for him. He says, come across, Bill, he says, there's two Irish men causing a bit of a disturbance. Aye, he says, I'll come across I: He was very big wasn't he? RP: So he—he goes across you know and these Irishmen sparring out with one another 'ere, what's the bother—outside, outside. They looked at him but they didn't seem to reach 'em—I said outside. And he gets hold of both of 'em. Bangs both of their heads together and pushes 'e, out. He were a big fellow you know

(continued)

(continued)

No.	D.O.B.	Gender	Location	Q. 1 Home brewing (HB)?	Q. 2 Parents drinking habits
105	1893	F	London	Mother made ginger beer and rhubarb wine—drunk by whole family	Father went to pub Sunday lunch times when he was not working
106	1887	M	Lancs	No HB	Did not say if father went to pub
107	1893	M	Liverpool	No HB	No pubs
108	1904	M	Liverpool	No HB	No pubs
109	1889	M	Liverpool	No HB	Father strict teetotaler
110	1889	M	Essex	See next column	*I*: Did she make wine? *AB*: Yes. Parsnip wine. Oh what's the name of it—sloe—sloe wine—sloe wine, sloe wine, sloe gin. All of us never drank it, nor did dad. Dad was teetotal and mother was a teetotaler. And—and—when—when I moved into that house and when dad died I threw—I threw away about a dozen bottles of different wine that was made—years and years old. Man'd stood on his head if he'd have drank it. They didn't half—the builder didn't half make a song about it too—because I threw it away *I*: Who'd have drunk it at the time—who did she make it for? *AB*: Used to give it away *I*: Used to give it to friends? *AB*: Yes. Some friends—one thing and another. 'Cos we were never—we were all teetotalers. We was all teetotalers 'til we left home anyhow. There was—there was only two—the oldest girl I think and the—and the brother that did have a drink but—the oldest brother and myself—I never touched it *I*: Never? *AB*: No
111	1892	F	Liverpool	Not asked	Father went to pub regularly. Mother was a 'staunch teetotaler'

(continued)

No.	D.O.B.	Gender	Location	Q. 1 Home brewing (HB)?	Q. 2 Parents drinking habits
112	1901	M	Guildford	No HB	Father went to pub occasionally. Mother teetotaler
113	1887	M	London	Brewed herb beer	*I:* Would he ever go out for a drink or something after he got home from work? *EP:* Oh yes, the pubs were open 'til twelve o'clock midnight then. And the other side the river they were open 'til half past twelve? *I:* Would he always go out when he came in the evening? *EP:* He'd have his supper first. And perhaps I'd be in bed and the—all the children. He might take mam out—just for—wouldn't be far to go, just round the corner. Have a bottle of Guinness
114	1892	F	Liverpool	No HB	*I:* Did either your granny or your mother have any interests at all outside the home? *MG:* No, nothing at all *I:* Did they ever go out to enjoy themselves at all? *MG:* No. Only—you know, for a glass of beer. Oh they'd go in—in—oh they'd enjoy that
115	1887	F	Liverpool	No HB	*I:* Never went to a pub or a club or anything like this? *AS:* No. No. No *I:* Did he drink? *AS:* No. He wasn't a teetotaler but he never—no. The only thing, before he died he longed for a glass of beer and I went up to Lark Lane to that place and I was terrified because I'd never been in the place before and I bought—mother told me to get two bottles of Whitbread's—and I got this, three of them. He only took a—just about that much off my—and he never bothered any more. It was just a fancy he had. Yes, just a fancy and he passed on just about a week afterwards so—yes. Yes
116	1895	F	Liverpool	No HB	Father went to pub
117	1893	F	Liverpool	Not asked	Not asked
118	1880	M	Lancs	No HB	Did not know if father went to pub

(continued)

(continued)

No.	D.O.B.	Gender	Location	Q. 1 Home brewing (HB)?	Q. 2 Parents drinking habits
119	1884	F	Liverpool	No HB	No pubs
120	1904	M	Liverpool	No HB	No pubs
121	1903	M	Liverpool	No HB	Father went to pub at weekends. Mother went occasionally
122	1895	M	Lancs	Mother made beer and tried to make stout	Not asked
123	1897	F	London	Mother made herb beer	Father strict teetotaler
124	1879	M	Essex	No HB	*I*: Can you remember anything you did with your mother or father on Christmas Day? *JT*: Well—when we got older—used to buy 'em something. I generally used to buy him a bottle of whisky. That's when we went to work you know. And a bottle of whisky only cost three bob then. Half a pint of beer was a penny. Half a pint of what they called porter was three farthings *I*: That was cheaper than beer? *JT*: Yes, it was a—I don't know what it was made of, it was a kind of mixture. You never hear of it now, porter
125	1878	F	Essex	No HB	Father went to pub occasionally
126	1895	F	London	No HB	Mother kept a four and a half gallon cask of beer for home consumption
127	1900	M	Manchester	Mother made mead	Not asked. Jewish family. Father member of Jewish working men's club. Travelled for business
128	1902	F	Yorkshire	Not asked	No pubs
129	1887	F	Colchester	Brewed beer	No pubs. Drank at home
130	1901	M	Wales	Mother made meth which was a sort of honey wine or mead	Not asked

(continued)

No.	D.O.B.	Gender	Location	Q. 1 Home brewing (HB)?	Q. 2 Parents drinking habits
362	1885	M	Edinburgh	No HB	Father strict teetotaler
363	1885	F	Dumfries	Made 'botanic beer'—non alcoholic	Father strict teetotaler
367	1886	M	Glasgow	No HB	Father was 'in the spirit line'—managing or working in pubs, unclear which. However father was a strict teetotaler
377	1890	F	Cardiff	Mother made small beer	Father teetotal—presumably 'small beer' was non-alcoholic?
378	1904	F	Edinburgh	Parents drank beer at home—not sure if HB	I: Did he ever go out to any pubs at all? MN: Yes I: Oh his own? MN: Yes I: Or did he go with friends? MN: Well he would go on his own or—or with friends. Occasionally—I mean—it would—a pint of beer or a half a pint of beer was all that he would go for, but he went into a pub I: Did he ever take your mother in with him? MN: Oh never. Oh—oh no. Oh she wouldn't have been seen dead in one

(continued)

(continued)

No.	D.O.B.	Gender	Location	Q. 1 Home brewing (HB)?	Q. 2 Parents drinking habits
382	1904	F	Dorset	No HB	EC: Father used to have a glass of beer occasionally but he never—used to get drunk or anything like that I: Did he go to the pub then? EC: Oh yes. Yes. Now my grandma—I tell you—when I was—how old was I—about twelve or thirteen I suppose—oh she must have been—must have been going on a long time before that, but I can particularly remember—you know they used to wear the capes, the old ladies, and a little bonnet with a—rose in the—or something in the front, and tied under the chin? Well she used to—put her cloak on, take her little jug, go down what is the St ar now, used to be the Prince of Wales. Go down there and get a—half a pint of stout. Go home, take her bit of cheese, and she used to go down to a friend's called Mrs Tizzard, Emma, we used to call her. And she used to take her—her bread and cheese and her half a pint of stout down there and have that there with Emma. And I can see her now. With her cloak and her little jug you know. No. No
435	1894	F	Dumfries	No HB	I: Was there any drinking at Christmas or New Year? AS: Any what? I: Drinking AS: Drinking, oh aye, they—they—they did—they—they could—well, whisky was on the go you know. But—the—it—it was chiefly tea you know, I mean it was tea—after that, tea to the dumpling and—and—and that I: What did your mother and father think about drink? AS: Oh they—my father—my father took whisky you see, mother didnae drink

(continued)

No.	D.O.B.	Gender	Location	Q. 1 Home brewing (HB)?	Q. 2 Parents drinking habits
207	1899	M	Shetlands	No HB	I: Did people drink on these occasions? JL: No, no, no, they didn't drink, no, no, they didn't—they didn't. You mean strong drink? I: I meant beer or whisky? JL: No, no, no, they—they—no, not—here again Feltar was rather took you a while to get that you see. There was nobody selled it you see. The merchants wasn't licensed to sell liquor, you see, that's the thing. Except they had a bit of on the sly about them you know. Yes, yes, yes, yes
233	1904	M	Isle Lewis	Made HB using treacle and yeast	Not asked about pubs
260	1891	M	Glasgow	No HB but father ran pubs	I: Did your mother ever go down to the pub with your father? RF: Not at all. She never served a customer in her life I: Did she ever go for a drink herself? RF: Never, she never took drink in her life. She never tasted—whisky in her life. Without—unless it was a doctor's order

Data Extracted from Edwardian Family Life Study

Source Thompson P. and Lummis T. *Family Life and Work Experience Before 1918, 1870–1973*. 7th Edition: Colchester: Essex: UK Data Archive: SN: 2000, 10.5255/UKDA-SN-2000: accessed May 2009

There are 140 samples in total: 1–130 selected as presented in the interview transcripts then 130–140 selected geographically to allow for regional variations

BIBLIOGRAPHY

Atherton W.F. 1931. *History of House Buchanan*: No Other Publication Information.

Bacon S. 1979. 'Alcohol Research Policy: The Need for an Independent Phenomenologically Oriented Field of Studies': *Journal of Studies of Alcohol*: 8:2: p. 26.

Bailey P. 2003. *Popular Culture and Performance in the Victorian City*: Cambridge: Cambridge University Press.

Barnard A. 1889. *Noted Breweries of Great Britain and Ireland*: Volume 1: London: Joseph Carlson.

Barrows S. and Room R. (eds.). 1992. *Drinking Behaviour and Belief in Modern Society*: Berkeley, CA: University of California Press.

Baudrillard J. 2003.'The Ideological Genesis of Needs', in (ed.) Clarke D.B., Doel M., and Housiaux K. *The Consumption Reader*: London: Routledge.

Beckingham D. 2010. 'An Historical Geography of Liberty: Lancashire and the Inebriates Acts': *Journal of Historical Geography*: 36:4: pp. 1–14.

Beeton I. 1861. *The Book of Household Management*: London: S.O. Beeton.

Berridge V. 2013. *Demons: Our Changing Attitudes to Alcohol, Tobacco and Drugs*: Oxford: Oxford University Press.

Best G. 1985. *Mid-Victorian Britain, 1851–75*: London: Fontana Press.

Bourdieu P. 1984/2010. *Distinction: A Social Critique of the Judgment of Taste*: London: Routledge.

Briggs A. 1985. *Wine for Sale: Victoria Wine and the Liquor Trade 1860–1984*: London: B.T. Batsford Ltd.

Burnett J. 1983. *Plenty and Want: A Social History of Diet in England from 1815 to the Present Day*: London: Methuen & Co Ltd.

Burns E. 1995. *Bad Whisky*: Glasgow: Balvag Books.

© The Editor(s) (if applicable) and The Author(s) 2018
T. Hands, *Drinking in Victorian and Edwardian Britain*,
https://doi.org/10.1007/978-3-319-92964-4

Cage R.A. (Ed.). 1987. *The Working Class in Glasgow 1750–1914*: Kent: Croom Helm.

Clarke D.B., Doel M., and Housiaux K. (eds.). 2003. *The Consumption Reader*: London: Routledge.

Corrigan P. 2011. *The Sociology of Consumption*: London: Sage.

Cowell F.R. 1974. *The Athenaeum: Club and Social Life in London 1824–1974*: London: Heinemann Education Books.

Curth L.H. 2003. 'The Medicinal Value of Wine in Early Modern England': *Social History of Alcohol and Drugs*: 18: pp. 35–50.

Davidoff L. 1986. *The Best Circles*: London: Croom Helm.

de Certeau M. 1984. *The Practice of Everyday Life*: Berkeley: University of California Press.

Dickens C. 1836/1996. *Sketches by Boz*: London: Penguin.

Dickens C. 1853. *Household Words*: Volume VIII: www.djo.org.uk/household-words/volume-viii-p: accessed 15/09/2014.

Dikotter F., Laarmann L., and Xun Z. 2004. *Narcotic Culture: A History of Drugs in China*: Chicago: Chicago University Press.

Donnachie I. 1979. *A History of the Brewing Industry in Scotland*: Glasgow: Bell & Bain.

Duis P. 1998. *The Saloon: Public Drinking in Chicago and Boston, 1880–1920*: Chicago: University of Illinois Press.

Fahey D. 1971. 'Temperance and the Liberal Party—Lord Peels' Report, 1899': *Journal of British Studies*: 10:2: pp. 132–159.

Foster T. 1990. *Pale Ale*: Boulder, CO: Brewers Publications.

Francatelli C. 1853/1977. *A Plain Cookery Book for the Working Classes*: London: Routledge.

Gately I. 2009. *Drink: A Cultural History of Alcohol*: New York: Gotham Books.

Girouard M. 1990. *Victorian Pubs*: New Haven, CT: Yale University Press.

Greenaway J. 2003. *Drink and British Politics Since 1830: A Study in Policy Making*: Basingstoke: Palgrave Macmillan.

Griffiths A.G.F. 1907. *Clubs and Clubmen*: London: Hutchinson.

Gusfield J. 1992. 'Benevolent Repression: Popular Culture, Social Structure and the Control of Drinking', in (eds.) Barrows S. and Room R. *Drinking Behaviour and Belief in Modern Society*: Berkeley, CA: University of California Press: pp. 76–91.

Gutzke D. 1989. *Protecting the Pub: Brewers and Publicans Against Temperance*: Suffolk: The Boydell Press.

Gutzke D. 2005. *Pubs and Progressives: Reinventing the Public House in England 1896–1960*: Chicago: Northern Illinois University Press.

Hames G. 2012. *Alcohol in World History*: London: Routledge.

Harrison B. 1971. *Drink and the Victorians: The Temperance Question in England 1815–1872*: London: Faber & Faber.

Heron C. 2003. *Booze: A Distilled History.* Toronto: Between the Lines.

Hill G. 1902. 'Bar and Saloon London', in (Ed.) Sims G.R. *Living London: It's Work and It's Play, It's Humour and It's Pathos, It's Sights and It's Scenes.* London: Cassell: pp. 286–288.

Hodgson B. 2011. *In the Arms of Morpheus: The Tragic History of Laudanum, Morphine and Patent Medicines.* Buffalo, NY: Firefly Books.

Houghland J.E. 2014.'The Origins and Diaspora of the IPA', in (eds.) Patterson M. and Hoalst-Pullen N. *The Geography of Beer: Regions, Environment & Societies.* New York: Springer: pp. 119–131.

Jacobs Soloman L. 2012. *Gin: A Global History.* London: Reakton Books.

Johnstone G. 1996. 'From Vice to Disease? The Concepts of Dipsomania and Inebriety 1860–1908': *Social and Legal Studies.* 5:37: pp 37–56.

Klein R. 1993. *Cigarettes Are Sublime*: London: Duke University Press.

Knox W.W. 1999. *Industrial Nation: Work, Culture and Society in Scotland 1800–Present:* Edinburgh: Edinburgh University Press.

Maloney P. 1993. *Scotland and the Music Hall 1850–1914*: Manchester: Manchester University Press.

Manchester C. 2008. *Alcohol and Entertainment Licensing Laws.* London: Routledge-Cavendish.

May C. 1997. 'Habitual Drunkards and the Invention of Alcoholism 1800–1850': *Addiction Research.* 5:2: pp. 56–69.

Mayhew H. 1851/2008. *London Labour and the London Poor.* London: Bibliophile Books.

McCandless P. 1984. 'Curses of Civilisation: Insanity and Drunkenness in Victorian Britain': *British Journal of Addiction.* 79: pp. 49–58.

Meacham S. 1977. *A Life Apart: The English Working Class 1890–1914*: London: Thames & Hudson.

Milne-Smith A. 2011. *London Clubland: A Cultural History of Gender and Class in Late Victorian Britain*: London: Palgrave Macmillan.

Mitchell S. 1991. *Daily Life in Victorian England*: Westport: Greenwood Press.

Mitchell T. 2004. *Intoxicated Identities: Alcohol Power in Mexican History and Culture*: London: Routledge.

Nicholls J. 2011. *The Politics of Alcohol*: Manchester: Manchester University Press.

Owen C. 1992. *The Greatest Brewery in the World: A History of Bass, Ratcliff and Gretton*: Chesterfield: Derbyshire Record Society.

Paul H. 2001. *Bacchic Medicine: Wine and Alcohol Therapies from Napoleon to the French Paradox*: Amsterdam: Editions Rodopi.

Powers M. 1998. *Faces Along the Bar: Lore and Order in the Workingmen's Saloon, 1870–1920*: Chicago: University of Chicago Press.

Reinarz J. 2007. 'Promoting the Pint: Ale and Advertising in Late Victorian and Edwardian England': *Social History of Alcohol and Drugs.* 22:1: pp. 26–44.

Reinarz J. and Wynter R. 2016. 'The Spirit of Medicine: The Use of Alcohol in Nineteenth Century Medical Practice', in (eds.) Schmid S. and Schmidt-Haberkamp B. *Drink in the Eighteenth and Nineteenth Centuries*: London: Routledge.

Roman P.M. (Ed.). 1991. *The Development of Sociological Perspectives on Alcohol Use and Abuse*: Bruswick, NJ: Alcohol Research Documentation.

Rowntree S. 1908. *Poverty: A Study of Town Life*: London: MacMillan.

Sims G.R. (Ed.). 1902. *Living London: It's Work and It's Play, It's Humour and It's Pathos, It's Sights and It's Scenes*: London: Cassell.

Spiller B. 1984. *The Chameleon's Eye: James Buchanan & Company Limited 1884–1984*: London and Glasgow: James Buchanan.

The Pub and the People: A Worktown Study by Mass Observation: 1943: London: Victor Gollancz.

Townsend B. 2011. *Scotch Missed: Scotland's Lost Distilleries*: Glasgow: Neil Wilson Publishing.

Valverde M. 1998. *Diseases of the Will: Alcohol and the Dilemmas of Freedom*: Cambridge: Cambridge University Press.

Veblen T. 1889/1994. *The Theory of the Leisure Class*: New York: Dover Publications.

Warner J.H. 1980. 'Physiological Theory and Therapeutic Explanation in the 1860s: The British Debate on the Medical Use of Alcohol: *Bulletin of the History of Medicine*: 54:2: pp. 235–257.

Waugh A. 1957. *Merchants of Wine*: London: Cassel.

Weir R.B. 1974. 'The Distilling Industry in Scotland in the Nineteenth and Early Twentieth Centuries': PhD Dissertation: 2 Volumes: Edinburgh University.

Weir R.B. 1982. 'Distilling and Agriculture': *Agricultural History Review*: 32:1: pp. 49–62.

Weir R.B. 1984. 'Obsessed with Moderation: The Drink Trades and the Drink Question 1870–1930': *British Journal of Addiction*: 79: pp. 93–107.

Wilkinson F.A. n.d. *The Story of the Western Club: From Its Inception in 1825 to the Year 1900*: Booklet Written by a Member of the Western Club Glasgow.

Wilson R.G. 1998. 'The Changing Taste for Beer in Victorian Britain', in (eds.) Wilson R.G. and Gourvish T.R. *The Dynamics of the International Brewing Industry Since 1800*: London: Routledge: pp. 93–105.

Wilson R.G. and Gourvish T.R. (eds.). 1998. *The Dynamics of the International Brewing Industry Since 1800*: London: Routledge.

Woodbridge G. 1978. *The Reform Club, 1836–1974: A History of the Club's Records*: New York: The Reform Club.

Zheng Y. 2005. *The Social Life of Opium in China*: Cambridge: Cambridge University Press.

INDEX

A

B

© The Editor(s) (if applicable) and The Author(s) 2018
T. Hands, *Drinking in Victorian and Edwardian Britain*,
https://doi.org/10.1007/978-3-319-92964-4